Founded in 1876,. **Caixa Geral de Depósitos (CGD)** *is a financial institution which for several decades has been playing an important role in the development of national economy.*

Within the current historical cycle dominated by European integration **CGD** *is still a pioneer in the opening of new ways to the future.*

Caixa Geral de Depósitos *is a* **referral institution** *within the Portuguese financial market, a characteristic that implies the assembling of its best traditional values - rigour, transparency and balance - with a leading attitude as to the present changes and the future.*

Under the perspective of rendering a global and integrated financial service to the client, **Caixa Geral de Depósitos Group** *completes and enlarges the nature of a universal bank that the mother institution is clearly assuming.*

On the o... **Group co**... *in specif*... *the rende*... *such as:*... *Seguros F*......, **holding** *(Caixa-Participações, SGPS),* **leasing** *(Locapor and Imoleasing),* **factoring** *(lusofactor),* **fund management** *(Fundimo, Caixagest, etc.),* **venture capital** *and* **real estate.**

The **CGD Group** *- the largest Portuguese financial Group - gears its activity towards the development and search of new products and services in view of rendering a global and integrated service to its clients.*

On the other hand, the increasing of the nature of a universal bank provides a more accurate answer to the dynamics of the Portuguese economy internationalisation through the physical presence in other markets.

G000141588

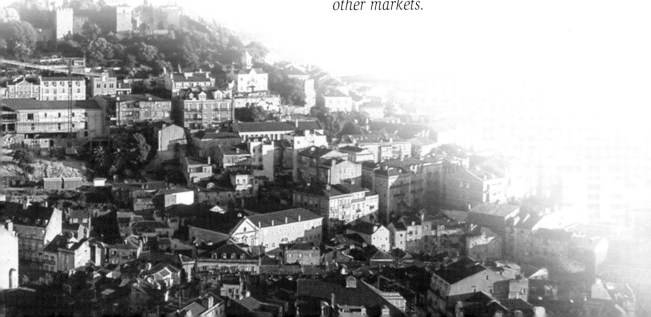

Following this strategic line of internationalisation **Caixa Geral de Depósitos** works in **Spain** with its affiliated banks Banco Luso Español, Banco de Extremadura and Banco Siméon.

It is also represented in **France** through its Paris Branch and the Banque Franco Portugaise (also present in **Monaco**), which develop their activity in close articulation with the Portuguese communities living in that country.

In **Luxembourg Caixa Geral de Depósitos** is represented through its Luxembourg Branch and in **Cape Verde** through its Cape Verde Branch.

In **Brazil, CGD** has also an affiliated bank, the Banco Financial Português and recently it acquired a new bank, the Banco Bandeirantes.

In **Mozambique, CGD** is represented through an affiliated bank, the Banco Comercial e de Investimentos.

It has also a Madeira Offshore Branch and it is present through its own representation offices in **Germany and Switzerland,** and through the Banco Simeón in **Venezuela** and **Mexico**.

Caixa Geral de Depósitos also plays an important role in the social and cultural development. In furthering its traditional programmes, **CGD** organizes a large number of initiatives of interest to Portuguese society in the intelectual, artistic, educational, scientific research, social welfare and sporting areas.

Culturgest, the **CGD GROUP** company specialising in cultural activities is the principal agency used and its schedules provide the public with a broad range of cultural events.

CGD works closely with the most representative Associations and Foundations performing significant actions in the field of social services and is the sponsor of many youth promotion programmes in sporting events.

CGD is also the sponsor of some of the most important initiatives promoted in the field of science and scientific research.

In this area, special reference shall be made to the important activities promoted in the last years by the **Portuguese Menopause Society** and the **European Menopause Society** with the participation of **Caixa Geral de Depósitos**.

MENOPAUSE AND THE HEART

MENOPAUSE AND THE HEART

Proceedings of an International Symposium organized by the
PORTUGUESE MENOPAUSE SOCIETY

Edited by

M. Neves-e-Castro, MD
Reproductive Medicine Clinic, Lisbon, Portugal

and

M. Birkhäuser, MD
University of Berne, Switzerland

T. B. Clarkson, MD
Wake Forest University, NC, USA

P. Collins, MD
National Heart and Lung Institute, London, UK

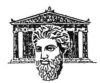

The Parthenon Publishing Group
International Publishers in Medicine, Science & Technology

NEW YORK   LONDON

Library of Congress Cataloging-in-Publication Data

Menopause and the heart : proceedings of an
  international symposium organized by the Portuguese
  Menopause Society / edited by M. Neves-e-Castro . . .
  [et al.].
         p. cm.
      Proceedings of the First International Symposium
  on Estrogens and the Cardiovascular System held in
  Estoril, Portugal.
      Includes bibliographical references and index.
      ISBN 1-85070-071-0
      1. Estrogen – Therapeutic use – Congresses
  2. Menopause – Hormone therapy – Congresses.
  3. Heart – Diseases – Hormone therapy – Congresses.
  4. Menopause – Complications – Prevention –
  Congresses.   5. Heart diseases in women –
  Congresses.   6. Heart – Diseases – Sex factors –
  Congresses.   I. Neves-e-Castro, M. (Manuel)
  II. Portuguese Menopause Society.   III. International
  Symposium on Estrogens and the Cardiovascular
  System (1st: 1998 : Estoril, Portugal)
      [DNLM: 1. Estrogen Replacement Therapy
  congresses.   2. Cardiovascular Diseases – prevention
  & control congresses.   3. Estrogens – physiology
  congresses.   WP 522 M547 1999]
  RC684.E75M46   1999
  616.1–dc21
  DNLM/DLC
  for Library of Congress   98-32248
                                                  CIP

British Library Cataloguing in Publication Data

Menopause and the heart : proceedings of an
  international symposium organized by the Portuguese
  Menopause Society
  1. Menopause – Hormone therapy – Congresses
  2. Heart – Diseases – Hormone therapy – Congresses
  I. Neves-e-Castro, M. II Portuguese Menopause Society
  616.1'2'061

  ISBN 1-85070-071-0

Published in the USA by
The Parthenon Publishing Group Inc.
One Blue Hill Plaza
PO Box 1564, Pearl River,
New York 10965, USA

Published in the UK and Europe by
The Parthenon Publishing Group Limited
Casterton Hall, Carnforth,
Lancs., LA6 2LA, UK

Copyright 1999 © Parthenon Publishing Group

First published 1999

Typeset by H&H Graphics, Blackburn, Lancs.
Printed and bound by Bookcraft (Bath) Ltd.,
Midsomer Norton, UK

Contents

List of principal contributors

M. Birkhäuser
Division of Gynecological Endocrinology
Department of Obstetrics and Gynecology
University of Berne
Schanzeneckstrasse 1
CH-3012 Berne
Switzerland

T.B. Clarkson
Comparative Medicine Clinical Research
   Center
Wake Forest University School of Medicine
Medical Center Boulevard
Winston-Salem, NC 27157-1040
USA

P. Collins
Division of Cardiac Medicine
Imperial College School of Medicine
National Heart and Lung Institute
Dovehouse Street
London SW3 6LY
UK

P.M. da Silva
Arterial Investigation Unit
Serviço de Medicina
Santa Marta Hospital
Rua de Santa Marta
1150 Lisbon
Portugal

B. de Lignieres
Department of Endocrinology and
   Reproductive Medicine
Hospital Necker
149 Rue de Sevres
75743 Paris Cedex 15
France

D. de Ziegler
Department of Obstetrics and Gynecology
Reproductive Endocrinology and Infertility
Zone Hospital
CH-1260 Nyon
Switzerland

J.M. Foidart
Department of Obstetrics and Gynecology
University of Liége
Hospital de la Citadelle
Bd du 12eme de Ligne, 1
B-4000 Liége
Belgium

F. Grodstein
Department of Medicine
Channing Laboratory
Brigham Women's Hospital
Harvard Medical School
181 Longwood Avenue
Boston, Massachusetts 02115
USA

J. Haarbo
Center for Clinical and Basic Research
Ballerup Byvej 222
DK-2750 Ballerup
Denmark

J. Lopo Tuna
UTIC-Arsénio Cordeiro
Santa Maria Hospital
Av. Prof. Egas Moniz
1600 Lisbon
Portugal

M. Massonneau
IöDP
107 rue Monge
75005 Paris
France

T. Mikkola
Department of Obstetrics and Gynecology
Helsinki University Central Hospital
Haartmaninkatu 2
FIN-00290 Helsinki
Finland

M. Neves-e-Castro
Reproductive Medicine Clinic
Av. Antonio Augusto Aguiar
24-2 D
1050 Lisbon
Portugal

A. Pines
Department of Medicine "T"
Ichilov Hospital
6 Weizman Street
Tel-Aviv 64239
Israel

G.M.C. Rosano
Department of Cardiology
Istitute H San Raffaele
Via Elio Chianesi, 33
00144 Rome
Italy

R. Sitruk-Ware
Department of Endocrinology
St. Antoine Hospital
184 rue du Fg Saint-Antoine
75012 Paris
France

S.O. Skouby
Department of Obstetrics and Gynecology
Frederiksberg Hospital
University of Copenhagen
DK-2000 Copenhagen F
Denmark

E. Wight
Department of Obstetrics and Gynecology
University Hospital Zurich
Frauenklinikstrasse 10
CH-8091 Zurich
Switzerland

Foreword

The management of the climacteric syndrome has become, within the last decade, an important subject, both for women and physicians. Women have become aware that most of the distressing symptoms that are often associated with the perimenopausal years can be prevented with proper hormonal replacement therapy (HRT). Physicians, in turn, have obtained evidence that HRT, besides its effects in symptom relief, is also effective in the prevention of osteoporosis and cardiovascular diseases(CVD).

Sex steroids seem, more and more, to display, by genomic and non-genomic mechanisms, pharmacological properties that are similar to those of many conventional drugs used by cardiologists. This is probably why HRT has marked effects not only in the primary prevention but also in the secondary prevention of the cardiovascular problems which are more prevalent in postmenopausal women.

No drug is devoid of side-effects, which mainly occur when it is administered for long periods of time, or for life. This is precisely the case with estrogenic and progestogenic steroids. Some epidemiological studies suggest an association of HRT, when used for longer than ten years, with a slight increase in the morbidity of breast cancer. This finding caused concern among women and physicians, regarding the best policy to follow and the selection of women who should and should not be put on long-term HRT. Cancer is a frightening disease for every woman, however, physicians should be careful when

they are called to put it into the perspective of long-term overall risks. Ten times more women die of CVD than of breast cancer, however HRT reduces the risk of dying from CVD by half. The balance of risk/benefits of HRT in relation to death is clearly favorable to HRT since the net number of lives saved is far superior to those lost, as confirmed by many studies.

In view of the importance of CVD for the menopausal woman, the Portuguese Menopause Society organised an International Symposium on 'Estrogens and the Cardiovascular System'. The contributors who kindly agreed to share their knowledge are amongst the top investigators to whom we owe much of the important information now available in this field.

We hope that this book 'Menopause and the Heart' will become an important reference used by cardiologists, internists, gynecologists and by all those interested in the prevention of disease and the preservation and promotion of the health of middle-aged women.

We are particularly grateful to our main sponsor Caixa Geral de Depósitos, for making both the Symposium and this publication possible. We are also indebted to The Parthenon Publishing Group for accepting to publish this book with enthusiasm and trust.

Manuel Neves-e-Castro, MD
President of the Portuguese Menopause Society
Vice-President of the European Menopause and Andropause Society

Vascular effects of estrogens 1

E. Wight, M. Barton, E. Espinosa, M. Tschudi, U. Arnet, Z. Yang and T.F. Lüscher

Epidemiological studies have demonstrated that the female hormone estrogen exerts profound vascular effects, especially with respect to the primary and secondary prevention of cardiovascular disease[1-4]. Estrogens have been shown to affect cardiac risk factors favorably, i.e. to improve dyslipidemia, carbohydrate metabolism and insulin sensitivity, and to reduce blood pressure and plasma fibrinogen levels[5]. In addition, estrogens augment or restore the endothelium-dependent vasodilatation in atherosclerotic blood vessels by increasing the local concentration of nitric oxide (NO)[6,7]. This is caused either by inducing nitric oxide synthase (NOS) activity[8] or by inhibiting NO degradation, as estrogens are potent antioxidants[9].

The influences of estrogens on the vascular wall seem to be exerted mainly in two ways[10]. One is through gene modulation mediated by the estrogen receptor(s), which have been identified on endothelial and vascular smooth muscle cells[11-13]. Secondly, a direct influence of estrogens is postulated, which may be the result of post-translational modifications of enzymes. While gene modulation typically results in long-term effects, direct steroid actions can rapidly influence vascular function. Recently, besides the influences of sex steroids on cardiovascular risk factors, these direct effects of estrogen on the blood vessel wall have gained much interest in cardiovascular research.

Vascular endothelial cells play an important role in regulation of vasomotion and maintenance of vascular structural integrity by balanced release of relaxing factors (NO, prostacyclin (PGI_2), endothelium-derived hyperpolarizing factor (EDHF)) and contracting factors (thromboxane A_2 (TXA_2),

prostaglandin H_2 (PGH_2), endothelin-1 (ET-1)) as well as growth promoters (basic fibroblast growth factor (bFGF), platelet derived growth factor (PDGF), ET-1) and inhibitors (NO, heparin, transforming growth factor beta (TGFβ)) (Figure 1)[14,15].

Treatment of rats with 17β-estradiol enhances NOS mRNA expression and enzyme activity in vascular and non-vascular tissue from both females and males (Figure 2)[8].

In the uterine artery of the rat, endothelium-dependent relaxations, induced by acetylcholine, correlate with the serum concentration of estradiol in young, pregnant, middle-aged (9–12 months of age) and ovariectomized rats[16].

In situ measurement of endothelial NO release, stimulated by calcium ionophore, showed in the aorta but not in the pulmonary artery of aged rats (33 months of age) a decreased liberation of NO compared to young (5 to 6 months of age) controls[17]. Furthermore, endothelium-dependent relaxations of aortal segments to calcium ionophore and acetylcholine *in vitro* correlated well to the directly measured NO release. The amount of detected NO from the aorta was unaffected by superoxide dismutase (SOD), suggesting that the reduced NO concentrations, measured in aged rats, were not caused by an enhanced oxidative degradation of the NO radical.

Pregnancy is a state of high NO availability in the uterine vasculature owing to up-regulation of NOS[18]. In the uterine vascular bed of pregnant rats near term, this leads to increased sensitivity (pD_2) to acetylcholine compared to non-pregnant controls, while maximum relaxations from this mediator were unaltered in both groups. Treating pregnant and non-pregnant animals

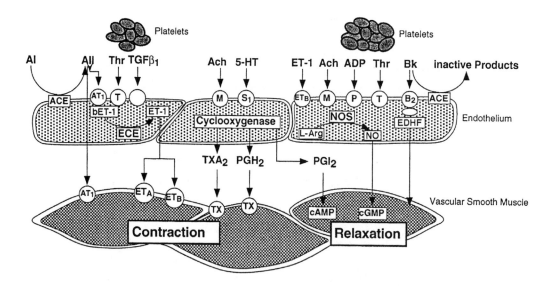

Figure 1 The endothelium releases both relaxing and contracting factors. The former include nitric oxide (NO), prostacyclin (PGI$_2$) and the endothelium-derived hyperpolarizing factor (EDHF). NO and PGI$_2$ not only cause relaxation of vascular smooth muscle cells via cyclic guanosine monophosphate (cGMP) and cyclic adenosine monophosphate (cAMP), respectively, but also inhibit platelet function. The contracting factors include the local renin–angiotensin system, endothelin-1 (ET-1) and cyclooxygenase-derived contracting factors such as thromboxane A$_2$ (TXA$_2$) and prostaglandin H$_2$ (PGH$_2$). In addition, the cyclooxygenase pathway is a source of oxygen-derived free radicals, which can inactivate NO. AI, angiotensin I; AII, angiotensin II; ACE, angiotensin converting enzyme; Ach, acetylcholine; ADP, adenosine diphosphate; Bk, bradykinin; bET, big-endothelin; ECE, endothelin converting enzyme; 5-HT, 5-hydroxytryptamine; TGFβ$_1$, transforming growth factor β$_1$; Thr, thrombin. Circles, receptors: AT$_1$, angiotensin receptor; B$_2$, bradykinin receptor; ET$_{A/B}$, endothelin $_{A/B}$ receptor; M, muscarinic receptor; P, purinic receptor; S$_1$, serotonin receptor; T, thrombin receptor; TX, thromboxane receptor

chronically with L-nitroarginine methylester (L-NAME), and thereby blocking the NOS, reduced maximum relaxation to acetylcholine only in non-pregnant rats, while leaving sensitivity and maximum response to this mediator unchanged in pregnant animals.

The sensitivity to sodium nitroprusside (SNP), which elicits endothelium-independent relaxations, on the other hand, is diminished in pregnancy compared to non-pregnant controls, as evidenced by a reduced pD$_2$ value. Again, this result is in accordance with NOS up-regulation during pregnancy, as the NO donor SNP meets high local NO concentrations. L-NAME medication during pregnancy increases sensitivity to SNP and brings pD$_2$ levels back to values seen in non-pregnant controls[16].

Besides having an effect on the release of NO, estrogens up-regulate serum levels of prostacyclin[19], which, like NO, is a vasodilator and inhibits platelet aggregation. In addition, estrogens are able to inhibit endothelin production, reducing its contractile effects (Figure 2)[20,21]. A recently published study demonstrated that estrogens promote human endothelial cell attachment on extracellular matrix components and stimulate endothelial cell migration and proliferation[22]. This process may be of importance in the repair of endothelial injuries and with respect to angiogenesis.

Besides enhancing endothelium-dependent, mediator-operated vasodilatation[23], estrogens also exert direct and endothelium-independent relaxing effects on vascular smooth muscle cells (VSMCs), most likely via blockade of Ca^{2+} channels (Figure 2)[24,25].

In premenopausal women, the estrogen receptor expression is inversely correlated

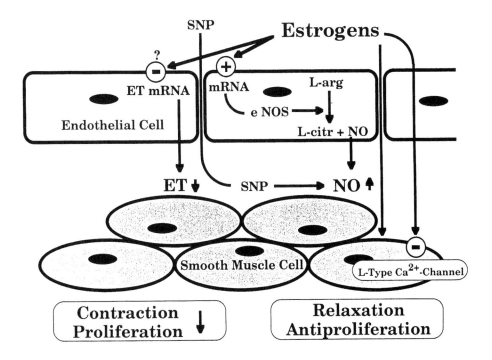

Figure 2 Effects of estrogens on the vascular wall. Estrogens induce nitric oxide (NO) synthase expression in endothelial cells (eNOS mRNA) and therefore enhance vascular NO release via the L-arginine–L-citrulline pathway. NO leads to relaxation in the underlying vascular smooth muscle cells and inhibits migration and proliferation, besides blocking thrombocyte aggregation. In addition, estrogens enhance prostacyclin synthesis and inhibit endothelin (ET)-1 production by endothelial cells. Furthermore, estrogens exhibit proliferative and migratory influences on endothelial cells, in contrast to their influences on vascular smooth muscle cells. Estrogens, besides influencing vascular smooth muscle cells indirectly through endothelial mediators, can also directly exert a relaxing effect on the muscle layer, probably via blockade of calcium channels. Sodium nitroprusside (SNP) causes vasodilatation by releasing NO

with atherosclerosis in coronary arteries, strongly indicating a functional role for estrogen in the cardiovascular system[26]. Proliferation and migration of VSMCs are believed to contribute importantly to intimal thickening in atherosclerosis, restenosis after transluminal angioplasty and venous bypass graft disease[27–29]. However, the effects of estrogens on VSMCs are still controversial, as different studies have found inhibiting or enhancing influences on proliferation, depending on the species or the vascular bed examined[30–32]. Yet, in humans it was clearly demonstrated that 17β-estradiol inhibits cell proliferation and migration in response to PDGF and bFGF in VSMCs of postmenopausal women and also of age-matched men with

coronary artery disease (Figure 2)[33,34]. Likewise, estrogens are able to inhibit neointimal proliferation after balloon injury in animal models[35].

CONCLUSION

Antiproliferative, antimigratory and direct vasodilating actions of estrogens on VSMCs may therefore contribute, together with the effects of estrogens on endothelial cells and cardiovascular risk factors, to the lower incidence of cardiovascular disease in premenopausal and postmenopausal women taking hormone replacement therapy compared to age-matched men.

References

1. Stampfer MJ, Colditz GA, Willett WC, *et al.* Postmenopausal estrogen therapy and cardiovascular disease. Ten-year follow-up from the Nurses' Health Study. *N Engl J Med* 1991;325:756–62

2. The Writing Group for the PEPI Trial. Effects of estrogen or estrogen/progestin regimens on heart disease risk factors in postmenopausal women. *J Am Med Assoc* 1995;273:199–208

3. Sullivan JM. Atherosclerosis and estrogen replacement therapy. *Int J Fertil* 1994;39(Suppl. 1):28–35

4. Gruchow HW, Anderson AJ, Barboriak JJ, *et al.* Postmenopausal use of estrogen and occlusion of coronary arteries. *Am Heart J* 1988;115:954–63

5. Rosano GMC, Chierchia SL, Leonardo F, *et al.* Cardioprotective effects of ovarian hormones. *Eur Heart J* 1996;17(Suppl D):15–19

6. Gilligan DM, Quyyumi AA, Cannon RO, *et al.* Effects of physiological levels of estrogen on coronary vasomotor function in postmenopausal women. *Circulation* 1994;89:2545–51

7. Gilligan DM, Badar DM, Panza JA, *et al.* Acute vascular effects of estrogen in postmenopausal women. *Circulation* 1994;90:786–91

8. Weiner CP, Lizasoain I, Bailis SA, *et al.* Induction of calcium-dependent nitric oxide synthases by sex hor-mones. *Proc Natl Acad Sci USA* 1994;91:5212–16

9. Katsuaki S, Shimosegawa Y, Nakano M. Estrogens as natural antioxidants of membrane phospho-lipid peroxidation. *FEBS Lett* 1987;210:37–9

10. Gorodeski GI, Utian WH. *Epidemiology and Risk Factors of Cardiovascular Disease in Postmenopausal Women.* New York: Raven Press, 1994

11. Colburn P, Buonassisi V. Estrogen-binding sites in endothelial cell cultures. *Science* 1978;201:817–19

12. Karas RH, Patterson BL, Mendelsohn ME. Human vascular smooth muscle cells contain functional estrogen receptor. *Circulation* 1994;89:1943–50

13. Inoue S, Hoshino SJ, Miyoshi H, *et al.* Identification of a novel isoform of estrogen receptor, a potential inhibitor of estrogen action, in vascular smooth muscle cells. *Biochem Biophys Res Commun* 1996;219:766–72

14. Lüscher TF, Vanhoutte PM. *The Endothelium: Modulator of Cardiovascular Function.* Boca Raton, FL: CRC Press, 1990

15. Lüscher TF. The endothelium in hypertension: bystander, target or mediator? *J Hypertens* 1994;12:S105–S116

16. Wight E, Küng CF, Moreau P, *et al.* Chronic blockade of nitric oxide synthase and endothelin receptors during pregnancy in the rat: effect on reactivity of the uterine artery *in vitro. J Soc Gynecol Invest* 1998;5:in press

17. Tschudi MR, Barton M, Bersinger NA, *et al.* Effect of age on kinetics of nitric oxide release in rat aorta and pulmonary artery. *J Clin Invest* 1996;98:899–905

18. Weiner CP, Knowles RG, Moncada S. Induction of nitric oxide synthases early in pregnancy. *Am J Obstet Gynecol* 1994;171:838–43

19. Mikkola T, Turunen P, Avela K, *et al.* 17-beta estradiol stimu-lates prostacyclin, but not endothelin-1, production in human vascular endothelial cells. *J Clin Endocrinol Metab* 1995;80:1832–6

20. Ylikorkala O, Orpana A, Puolakka J, *et al.* Postmenopausal hormonal replace-ment decreases plasma levels of endothelin-1. *J Clin Endocrinol Metab* 1995;80:3384–7

21. Polderman KH, Stehouver CDA, van Kamp GJ, *et al.* Influence of sex hormones on plasma endothelin levels. *Ann Intern Med* 1993;118:429–32

22. Morales DE, McGowan KA, Grant DS, *et al.* Estrogen promotes angiogenic activity in human umbilical vein endothelial cells *in vitro* and in a murine model. *Circulation* 1995;91:755–63

23. Mügge A, Riedel M, Barton M, *et al.* Endothelium-independent relaxation by 17β-oestradiol of human coronary arteries *in vitro. Cardiovasc Res* 1993;27:1939–42

24. Jiang C, Sarrel PM, Lindsay DC, *et al.* Endothelium-independent relaxation of rabbit coronary artery by 17β-oestradiol *in vitro. Br J Pharmacol* 1991;104:1033–7

25. Shu-Zhong H, Karaki H, Ouchi Y, *et al.* 17β-Estradiol inhibits Ca^{2+} influx and Ca^{2+} release induced by thromboxane A_2 in porcine coronary artery. *Circulation* 1995;91:2619–26

26. Losordo DW, Kearney M, Kim EA, *et al.* Variable expression of the estrogen receptor in normal and atherosclerotic coronary arteries of premenopausal women. *Circulation* 1994;89:1501–10

27. Ross R. The pathogenesis of atherosclerosis: a perspective for the 1990s. *Nature (London)* 1993;362:801–9

28. Yang Z, Stulz P, von Segesser L, *et al.* Different interactions of platelets with arterial and venous coronary bypass vessels. *Lancet* 1991;337:939–43

29. Lüscher TF, Diederich D, Siebenmann R, *et al.* Differences between endothelium-dependent

relaxation in arterial and in venous coronary bypass grafts. *N Engl J Med* 1988;319:462–7

30. Espinosa E, Oemar BS, Lüscher TF. 17β-Estradiol and smooth muscle cell proliferation in aortic cells of male and female rats. *Biochem Biophys Res Commun* 1996;221:8–14

31. Vargas R, Wroblewska B, Rego A, *et al.* Oestradiol inhibits smooth muscle cell proliferation of pig coronary artery. *Br J Pharmacol* 1993;109:612–17

32. Farhat MY, Vargas R, Dingaan B, *et al. In vitro* effect of oestradiol on thymidine uptake in pulmonary vascular smooth muscle cell: role of the endothelium. *Br J Pharmacol* 1992;107: 679–83

33. Yang Z, Julmy F, Mohadjer A, *et al.* 17β-Oestradiol inhibits growth of human vascular smooth muscle: similar effects in cells from females and males. *Eur Heart J* 1995;16:A1149

34. Dai-Do D, Espinosa E, Liu G, *et al.* 17β-Estradiol inhibits proliferation and migration of human vascular smooth muscle cells: similar effects in cells from postmenopausal females and in males. *Cardiovasc Res* 1996;32:980–85

35. Chen S-J, Li H, Durand J, *et al.* Estrogen reduces myointimal proliferation after balloon injury of rat carotid artery. *Circulation* 1996;93:577–84

Estrogen and the vessel wall: effects on endothelium-dependent stimuli

2

P.M. da Silva

INTRODUCTION

Cardiovascular disease, particularly coronary heart disease (CHD), is the main cause of death in women, being responsible for 14% of all deaths in women[1-3]. Stroke or myocardial infarction account for the death of one out of every two women after 50 years, surpassing by far the total number of deaths caused by cancer in women of this age[2].

However, white Caucasian premenopausal women present a lower cardiovascular risk, smaller than men in the same age group. After the menopause, the cardiovascular risk increases linearly and in parallel with that of the men, starting to converge in more advanced ages in such a way that the incidence of coronary disease in older age groups is very similar[4,5]. If we bear in mind that a woman has a life expectancy, on average, of 8 to 10 years more than a man, the absolute number of deaths related to cardiovascular disease in women exceeds that of men.

Recently, Sacks and colleagues[6,7] thoroughly reviewed the mechanisms by which sex hormones affect the lipoprotein metabolism. They reached the conclusion that estrogens are capable of increasing the production rate of large, triglyceride-rich very low-density lipoprotein (VLDL) particles, thus raising the plasma levels of total triglycerides. On the other hand, these hormones lower the low-density lipoproteins (LDL) levels by increasing the number of hepatic LDL receptors, and consequently the rate of LDL catabolism. Finally, estrogens could suppress hepatic triglyceride lipase activity, delay high-density lipoprotein (HDL) clearance and increase the HDL plasma levels[7] (Table 1).

During the menopause, the plasma levels of total cholesterol and LDL cholesterol, as well as total triglycerides, tend to increase whilst the plasma level of HDL cholesterol tends to decrease. As a result, a significant increase in the total cholesterol/HDL ratio occurs. These modifications in lipid profile are usually attributed, at least partially, to the loss of the protective effects of estrogen and justify the introduction of estrogen-replacement therapy in postmenopausal women.

The beneficial effects of estrogen replacement therapy on lipid levels have been well documented[8-10] and have been related to significant reductions in cardiovascular risk. In epidemiological studies, estrogen replacement therapy has reduced the risk of adverse coronary events by almost 50%, with the greatest beneficial effects in women with existing CHD[10,11].

Table 1 Effects of sex hormones on lipoprotein metabolism

	Progestin	Estrogen
VLDL		
Fractional catabolic rate	↑	↔
Production rate	↑ or ↓	↑↑
LDL		
Fractional catabolic rate	↑ or ↔	↑↑
Production rate	↓ or ↑ (?)	↑
HDL	↓ (?)	↑

↑ increased; ↓ decreased; ↔ no change. Estrogen increases the transcription rate of apoB mRNA, apoA-I mRNA and LDL receptor mRNA

However, the effects of sex hormones, particularly estrogens, on the lipid profile account for only 30–50% of the observed reduction in the risk of cardiovascular morbidity and mortality. Therefore, other additional factors (Table 2) have been suggested and studied in various animal models *in vivo* and *ex vivo* [11,12].

In our unit, we have started our studies in endothelial function by discussing the effects of estrogens on the endothelium in the modulation of blood vessel tone (and the maintenance of patency) in women.

MEASURING ENDOTHELIAL FUNCTION. NON-INVASIVE ASSESSMENT OF VASCULAR REACTIVITY

More than 15 years ago, Furchgott and Zawadzki[13] concluded that the vaso-dilatory response to acetylcholine in an *in vitro* preparation of preconstricted rabbit aortic strips depended on the existence of a normal endothelium. The foundations for studying endothelial function and its role in the control of vascular tone were set.

A large variety of *in vitro* or *in vivo* techniques have been used in the study of endothelial function. However, the ability of an intact endothelium to produce various vasoactive substances in response to physiological stimuli, of which shear stress is a good example, or to different pharmacological stimuli (e.g. thrombin, acetyl-

Table 2 Potential cardioprotective effects of estrogen

Modulation of lipoprotein metabolism
Changes in the endothelial and vascular smooth muscle cell function
   modulation of blood vessel tone
   maintenance of patency
Other potential effects in
   blood pressure
   fasting glucose and insulin levels
   prostaglandin production
   fibrinolysis
   plasma fibrinogen level
   calcium antagonist effect

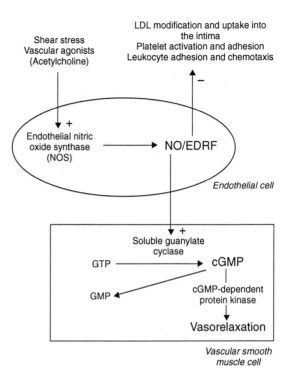

Figure 1 The nitric oxide/cGMP signal transduction system. NO, nitric oxide; EDRF, endothelium-derived relaxing factor

choline, metacholine, ADP) has been the foundation of the tests used for understanding the role of the endothelium in the control of local vascular tone and in the interaction between the vessel wall and platelets and leukocytes (Figure 1) [14].

The experimental methods *in vitro* have been widely discussed by Secombe and Schaff[15] and do not belong in this paper. On the other hand, the *in vivo* studies, owing to their invasive characteristics, have been limited to patients with symptoms of established vascular disease. In those studies, the endothelium-dependent changes in arterial diameter, usually evaluated by quantitative angiography, in response to vasoactive substances are compared with those obtained with endothelium-independent vasodilators (such as nitroglycerine or nitroprusside). Nevertheless, these techniques are not appropriate in the study of asymptomatic subjects or in a sequential evaluation of subjects who already have endothelial

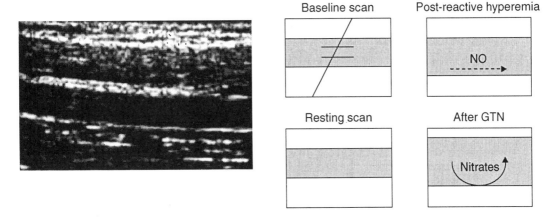

Figure 2 Graphic representation of a brachial vascular study. Diameter measurements are taken at the end of diastole on each scan and the percentage diameter change relative to the baseline vessel size is calculated. NO, nitric oxide; GTN, glyceryl trinitrate

dysfunction and various other diseases states, to whom eventually therapies to prevent the loss of NO/EDRF are given (L-arginine, antioxidants, HMG CoA reductase inhibitors, ACE inhibitors, or hormone replacement therapy in postmenopausal women).

In the meanwhile, Celermajer and colleagues[16,17] have developed a non-invasive test for studying endothelial function and vascular reactivity that is widely applicable, accurate and reproducible[18], and able to distinguish subjects with and without endothelial dysfunction. The method has been extensively described and discussed in reference 17. This technique requires an ultrasound scanner with a high-frequency linear transducer (7.5 MHz) with which the arterial diameter of a superficial artery can be evaluated (superficial femoral artery in children or brachial artery in adults). A resting scan is recorded and the baseline diameter of the target artery is compared with the diameter obtained after reactive hyperemia (endothelial-dependent flow-mediated vasodilatation) and after the administration of sublingual glyceryl trinitrate (GTN) spray (endothelial-independent vasodilatation) (Figure 2). It has been confirmed that the flow-dependent dilatation (FMD) of the human peripheral conduit arteries is mediated by NO (ERDF) and is attenuated or inhibited by the infusion of a NO synthase inhibitor, such as N^G-mono-methyl-L-arginine (L-NMMA)[19,20]. Reduced brachial artery FMD correlates closely with functional abnormalities of the coronary endothelium[21,22], and is associated with the presence of different major vascular risk factors and their interaction in subjects with asymptomatic endothelial dysfunction[23].

ESTROGENS, MENOPAUSE AND ENDOTHELIAL-DEPENDENT VASODILATATION

There is convincing evidence in animal models and in humans that estrogens could influence endothelial cell function and vasomotor tone. The acute administration of estradiol-17β reduces peripheral vascular resistance and improves coronary endothelium-dependent vasodilatation in response to acetylcholine in postmenopausal women[24-26].

It is well know that aging is one of the main determinants of vascular function. Aging *per se* alters the functional characteristics of endothelial cells. Celermajer and colleagues[27], using the non-invasive test of vascular reactivity, evaluated a possible relationship between endothelial function and aging and the different pattern of endothelial vasodilatation decline in men and women. It must be stressed that, of the 135 assessed women with no cardiovascular risk factors, 36 were postmenopausal and were not receiving hormone replacement therapy. It has been confirmed that the FMD decreased with age and developed in parallel with the differences in the patterns of cardiovascular morbidity and mortality already known between the sexes. The flow-dependent vasorelaxation was maintained in men until 41 years and declined after that at 0.21%/year; in women, the age-related decline began around 53 years, and subsequently decreased at a faster rate (0.49%/year; $p = 0.002$ compared with men). In face of these results and after confirming that the age at which endothelial dysfunction in women is evident coincided with the age of the physiological menopause, the authors[27] confirmed that this study supported a protective effect of estrogens on the endothelial cell and on vascular tone.

Curiously, Hashimoto and colleagues[28] have been able to confirm that the endothelium-dependent flow-mediated vasorelaxation varies during the menstrual cycle (they divided the menstrual cycle into the menstrual phase, the follicular phase and the luteal phase on the basis of the subjects' previous menstrual cycle, morning body temperature and actual menstruation, and confirmed these by serum concentrations of sex hormones) (Figure 3). These menstrual cycle-related vascular changes were independent of serum lipid profiles and blood pressure, and seemed to be dependent on serum estrogen levels. In conclusion, in this study the endogenous ovarian hormones, particularly estradiol, seemed to be involved in the menstrual cyclic variation of endothelium-dependent vasodilatation in healthy women.

The technical and functional characteristics of non-invasive assessment of FMD in the study of endothelial dysfunction make it easy to judge the importance of different therapeutic approaches to endothelial function. Lieberman and colleagues[29] studied, in a double-blind, placebo-controlled, cross-over

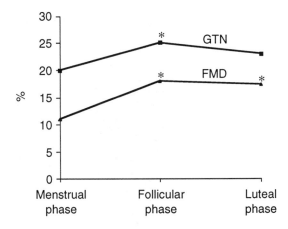

Figure 3 Effects of menstrual cycle on percentage increase in brachial artery diameter induced by flow-dependent dilatation (FMD) and glyceryl trinitrate (GTN). * $p < 0.01$ versus menstrual phase

trial, the impact of estrogen replacement therapy on brachial artery reactivity in postmenopausal women (average age, 55 ± 7 years) treated with a dose of 1 mg/day and 2 mg/day of oral estradiol during 9 weeks. The endothelium-dependent FMD of the brachial artery significantly improved in both treatment groups (percentage increase in brachial artery diameter induced by FMD of 13.5% and 11.6% for 1-mg and 2-mg doses, respectively, and of 6.8% for patients receiving placebo; $p < 0.05$ for each dose compared with placebo). In contrast, endothelium-independent responses to GTN were not significantly modified by estrogen replacement therapy (Figure 4).

CONCLUSION

These studies, using a non-invasive method to study vascular and endothelial function, point to a clear vasodilatory effect of estrogen in vascular reactivity. Estrogens could modulate the expression and transcription of different genes in the vascular wall and could also exert direct effects on arterial smooth muscle cells or stimulate the release of vasoactive substances. Mendelsohn and Karas[30] have recently suggested that the vasomotor effects of estradiol could be

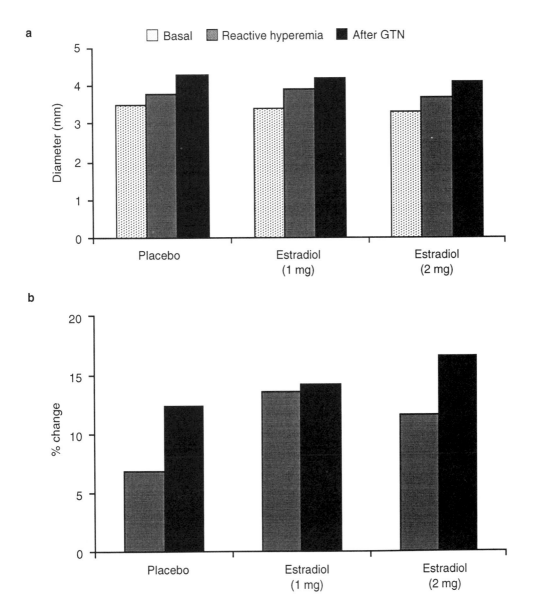

Figure 4 Effects of estradiol on brachial artery diameter (a) and percentage change (b) in postmenopausal women. GTN, glyceryl trinitrate

explained by the induction of EDRF/NO release, the antagonism of responses to endothelin-1 and hyperpolarization or calcium channel antagonism of vascular smooth muscle cells.

Future prospective and clearly designed studies are required to confirm the importance of these estrogen effects on vascular reactivity and to examine whether estrogen replacement therapy reduces cardiovascular mortality and morbidity as well as total mortality. The availability of a non-invasive assessment of vascular function allows endothelial dysfunction to be accepted as a surrogate endpoint in cardiovascular disease in postmenopausal women.

References

1. Kuhn FE, Rackley CE. Coronary heart disease in women. Risk factors, evaluation, treatment, and prevention. *Arch Intern Med* 1993;153:2626–36
2. American Heart Association. *Heart and Stroke Facts.* Dallas, Texas: American Heart Association, 1993
3. Fletcher JLM, Vessey MP. Coronary heart disease in women: current trends and health economics. In Birkhäuser MH, Rozenbaum H, eds. *European Consensus Development Conference on Menopause*, Montreux, Switzerland, September 1995. Paris: Éditions Eska, 1996:139–50
4. Castelli WP. Cardiovascular disease in women. *Am J Obstet Gynecol* 1988;158:1552–60
5. Lerner DJ, Kannel WB. Patterns in coronary heart disease – morbidity and mortality in sexes: a 26-year follow-up of the Framingham population. *Am Heart J* 1986;111:383–90
6. Sacks FM, Walsh BW. Sex hormones and lipoprotein metabolism. *Curr Opin Lipidol* 1994;5:236–40
7. Sacks FM, Gerhard M, Walsh BW. Sex hormones, lipoproteins, and vascular reactivity. *Curr Opin Lipidol* 1995;6:161–6
8. Kannel WB. Metabolic risk factors for coronary heart disease in women. Perspective from the Framingham Study. *Am Heart J* 1987;114;413–19
9. Walsh BW, Schiff I, Rosner B, *et al.* Effects of postmenopausal estrogen replacement on the concentrations and metabolism of plasma lipoproteins. *N Engl J Med* 1991;325:1196-204
10. Bush TL. Evidence for primary and secondary prevention of coronary artery disease in women taking estrogen replacement therapy. *Eur Heart J* 1996;17(Suppl D):9–14
11. Gerhard M, Ganz P. How do we explain the clinical benefits of estrogen? From bedside to bench [Editorial]. *Circulation* 1995;92:5–8
12. Rosano GMC, Chierchia SL, Leonardo F, *et al.* Cardioprotective effects of ovarian hormones. *Eur Heart J* 1996;17(Suppl D):15–19
13. Furchgott RF, Zawadzki JV. The obligatory role of endothelial cells in the relaxation of arterial smooth muscle by acetylcholine. *Nature (London)* 1980;288:373-6
14. Lloyd-Jones DM, Bloch KD. The vascular biology of nitric oxide and its role in atherogenesis. *Annu Rev Med* 1996;47:365–75
15. Seccombe JF, Schaff HV. *Vasoactive Factors Produced by the Endothelium: Physiology and Surgical Implications.* Austin: R. G. Landes Company (Medical Intelligence Unit), 1994:27–41

16. Celermajer DS, Sorensen KE, Gooch VM, *et al.* Non-invasive detection of endothelial dysfunction in children and adults at risk of atherosclerosis. Lancet 1992;340:1111–15
17. Sorensen K. Non-invasive assessment of endothelial function. In Vane JR, Born GVR, Welzel D, eds. *The Endothelial Cell in Health and Disease.* Stuttgart: Schattauer, 1995:183–98
18. Sorensen KE, Celermajer DS, Spielgelhalter DJ, *et al.* Non-invasive measurement of human endothelium dependent arterial responses: accuracy and reproducibility. *Br Heart J* 1995;74:247–53
19. Lieberman EH, Knab ST, Creager MA. Nitric oxide mediates the vasodilatation response to flow in humans (Abstract). *Circulation* 1994;90:I-138
20. Joannides R, Haefeli WE, Linder L, *et al.* Nitric oxide is responsible for flow-dependent dilatation of human peripheral conduit arteries *in vivo. Circulation* 1995;91:1314–19
21. Uehata A, Gerhard MD, Meredith IT, *et al.* Close relationship of endothelial dysfunction in coronary and brachial artery (Abstract). *Circulation* 1993;88:I-618
22. Anderson TJ, Uehata A, Gerhard MD, *et al.* Close relation of endothelial function in the human coronary and peripheral circulations. *J Am Coll Cardiol* 1995;26:1235–41
23. Celermajer DS, Sorensen KE, Bull C, *et al.* Endothelium-dependent dilation in the systemic arteries of asymptomatic subjects relates to coronary risk factors and their interaction. *J Am Coll Cardiol* 1994;24:1468–74
24. Gilligan DM, Badar DM, Panza JA, *et al.* Acute vascular effects of estrogen in postmenopausal women. *Circulation* 1994;90:786–91
25. Gilligan DM, Quyyumi AA, Cannon RO III. Effects of physiological levels of estrogen on coronary vasomotor function in postmenopausal women. *Circulation* 1994;89:2545–51
26. Reis SE, Gloth ST, Blumenthal RS, *et al.* Ethinyl estradiol acutely attenuates abnormal coronary vasomotor responses to acetylcholine in postmenopausal women. *Circulation* 1994;89:52–60
27. Celermajer DS, Sorensen KE, Spiegelhalter DJ, *et al.* Aging is associated with endothelial dysfunction in healthy men years before the age-related decline in women. *J Am Coll Cardiol* 1994;24:471–6
28. Hashimoto M, Akishita M, Eto M, *et al.* Modulation of endothelium-dependent flow-

mediated dilatation of the brachial artery by sex and menstrual cycle. *Circulation* 1995;92: 3431–5

29. Lieberman EH, Gerhard MG, Uehata A, *et al.* Estrogen improves endothelium-dependent, flow-mediated vasodilatation in postmenopausal women. *Ann Intern Med* 1994;121:936–41

30. Mendelsohn ME, Karas RH. Estrogen and the blood vessel wall. *Curr Opin Cardiol* 1994;9: 619–26

Estradiol and hormone replacement therapy: regulation of the vasoactive agents derived from human vascular endothelial cells

3

T. Mikkola

Coronary heart disease is the leading cause of morbidity and mortality in Western countries. Although women, during their reproductive years, are relatively well protected against occlusive vascular disorders, in postmenopausal women this protection rapidly ceases. Postmenopausal women have over 30% lifetime risk of dying of coronary heart disease, which is about ten times greater than the risk of dying of breast cancer or hip fractures. Moreover, a wide spectrum of cardiovascular complaints occur in these relatively young and active women. Therefore, prevention of cardiovascular disorders in postmenopausal women has great significance, because at least one-third of women's life is spent in the postmenopausal period.

ESTROGENS PROTECT AGAINST CARDIOVASCULAR DISORDERS

Cardiovascular health in fertile women is maintained, at least in part, by endogenous production of female sex steroids, particularly 17β-estradiol (E_2). This view is supported by the epidemiological finding that exogenous E_2 in hormone replacement therapy (HRT) also maintains vascular health (for review, see reference 1). However, the mechanisms whereby E_2 mediates this protection have remained largely unknown, because the E_2-induced long-term effects, e.g. favorable changes in blood lipids and lipoproteins, may account for only a part of the overall cardiovascular protection[2]. One of the most recent explanations involves the direct and relatively rapid effects of E_2 on the regulation of endothelial function, and in this context we briefly review this evidence.

VASCULAR ENDOTHELIUM

Endothelial cells cover the luminal surface of all blood vessels. It has been estimated that in a normal 70-kg adult, endothelial cells occupy a surface area of up to 1000 m^2, and weigh from 100 g to 1500 g. In the presence of a healthy vessel wall, platelet attachment and aggregation rarely occur, owing to the active role of endothelial cells, which provide an antithrombotic and anticoagulant surface for flowing blood. In addition to the obvious barrier and transport functions between the circulating blood and the underlying vessel wall, the endothelium influences its environment by the secretion of a wide range of biologically active factors. These include vasodilatory prostacyclin (PGI_2) and nitric oxide (NO), as well as vasoconstrictive endothelin-1 (ET-1)[3]. The balance between the endothelium-derived vasoactive factors may play a key role in the physiology of blood vessels and the pathogenesis of vascular diseases.

ESTRADIOL STIMULATES PROSTACYCLIN PRODUCTION IN ENDOTHELIAL CELLS

Prostacyclin production was markedly lower in the uterine arteries of postmenopausal women when compared to those of

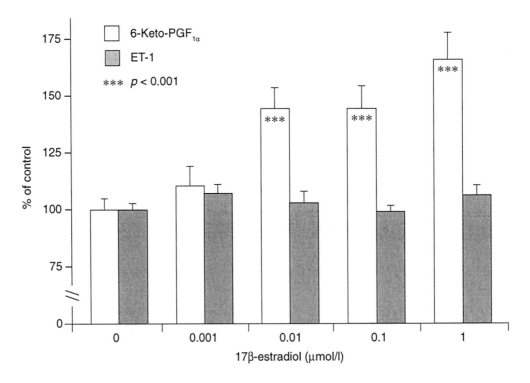

Figure 1 Effects of 17β-estradiol on 6-keto-prostaglandin(PG)F$_{1\alpha}$ and endothelin-1 (ET-1) production. Cultured HUVECs were incubated for 12 h without (control) or with the concentration indicated of estradiol in serum-free culture media. Statistical significances calculated against control. From Mikkola *et al.*, 1995[5]

premenopausal women, suggesting that vascular PGI$_2$ production may decrease concomitantly with the onset of menopause, and with the appearance of hypoestrogenism[4]. To evaluate the role of the endothelium, we used cultured human umbilical vein endothelial cells (HUVECs) to study the effect of E$_2$ on PGI$_2$ production. With these cells, E$_2$ (0.01–1 μmol/l) significantly increased PGI$_2$ production up to 66% (Figure 1)[5]. This stimulation was blocked in a dose-dependent manner by antiestrogenic tamoxifen (Figure 2). The E$_2$-induced stimulation of PGI$_2$ production could, however, be demonstrated only in the cells that were incubated in serum-free conditions, which may reveal the reason for the lack of the effect of E$_2$ in some earlier studies[6] in which serum was present. Moreover, E$_2$ stimulated PGI$_2$ production slowly, within hours, which might explain why others[7], by using only 5-min incubation, failed

to demonstrate the effect of E$_2$ on PGI$_2$ synthesis even in serum-free conditions.

In cultured HUVECs the concentration of E$_2$ (0.01 μmol/l) needed to stimulate PGI$_2$ production was considerably higher than that which exists physiologically or during HRT[5]. However, a 100-times lower E$_2$ concentration (physiological concentration) stimulated PGI$_2$ production in freshly harvested HUVECs[8]. This stimulation was blocked by tamoxifen. Because endothelial cells may lose some of their inherent functions in long-term culture[9], freshly harvested human vascular endothelial cells may better represent the *in vivo* situation than do cells passaged further[10,11].

In the experiments with cultured HUVECs[5] we also measured the release of ET-1. Estradiol had no effect on the release of ET-1 in any of these experiments. Therefore, apparently mechanisms other than solely a rise in plasma E$_2$ are responsible for the decreased

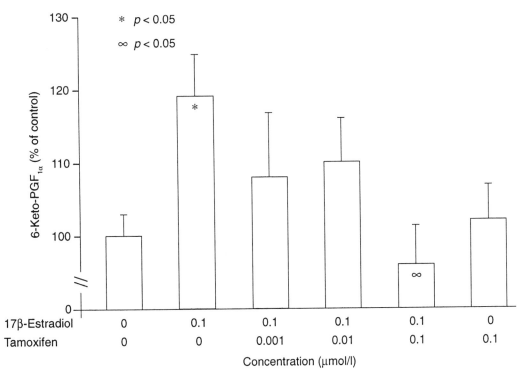

Figure 2 Effects of 17β-estradiol and tamoxifen separately or as incubated together on 6-keto-prostaglandin(PG)$F_{1\alpha}$ production. Cultured HUVECs were incubated for 12 h without (control) or with the concentration indicated of estradiol and/or tamoxifen in serum-free culture media. Statistical significance calculated against control (*) and against 0.1 μmol/l estradiol (∞). From Mikkola et al., 1995[5]

circulating ET-1 levels in postmenopausal women during the use of transdermal HRT[12].

ESTRADIOL AND NITRIC OXIDE

It has been demonstrated that E_2 induces the expression of constitutive nitric oxide synthase in human endothelial cells[13,14], whereas in bovine aortic endothelial cells E_2 enhanced NO production in some[15] but not all studies[16]. We found no effect of E_2 on the maximal activity of calcium-dependent NO production in cultured HUVECs[8]. It is possible that the use of different methods, which assess different aspects of NO production, could partly explain why E_2 enhanced endothelial cell NO production in some[13–15] but not all studies[8,16].

In vivo acute administration of E_2 transiently potentiated acetylcholine-stimulated vasodilatation in postmenopausal women[17], but this effect vanished after 3 weeks of transdermal E_2 administration[18]. Furthermore, sublingual E_2 increased blood flow and reduced resistance in the forearm of postmenopausal women[19]. Both these results were interpreted to indicate that E_2 could rapidly induce NO production *in vivo*.

HORMONE REPLACEMENT THERAPY INCREASES THE CAPACITY OF PLASMA TO STIMULATE PROSTACYCLIN PRODUCTION IN ENDOTHELIAL CELLS

In vivo, endothelial cells are flushed by circulating plasma (not by serum). Since plasma can stimulate PGI_2 and ET-1 production in endothelial cells[20], we studied whether the use of HRT is accompanied by changes in the capacity of plasma to direct

PGI_2 and/or ET-1 production in cultured HUVECs. Plasma samples were collected from 13 postmenopausal women before and after 6 months' use of oral HRT (Trisekvens, Novo Nordisk, Copenhagen, Denmark), and this plasma was added at 10% concentration to cultured HUVECs. HRT enhanced the ability of plasma to stimulate PGI_2 production by $21 \pm 6\%$ during the E_2 + norethisterone acetate phase and tended to do so also during the E_2-only phase ($11 \pm 10\%$), but caused no change in ET-1 release[21]. These data imply that the use of oral HRT triggers such beneficial changes in plasma, possibly protecting against the risk of cardiovascular disorders. It is conspicuous that this benefit was most marked during the use of the combined phase of HRT,

although the addition of progestin to HRT has been thought to be harmful with regard to cardiovascular protection[22].

CONCLUDING REMARKS

The acuteness of E_2-induced vascular changes strongly imply that one target for E_2 could indeed be the endothelium. This hypothesis is supported by a large volume of experimental data, as briefly reviewed above. It remains to be seen how large a proportion of HRT-induced protection against cardiovascular disorders is due to the beneficial effect of HRT on the endothelium.

References

1. Lobo RA, Speroff L. International consensus conference on postmenopausal hormone therapy and the cardiovascular system. *Fertil Steril* 1994;62(Suppl. 2):176S–179S

2. Walsh BW, Schiff I, Rosner B, *et al.* Effects of postmenopausal estrogen replacement on the concentrations and metabolism of plasma lipoproteins. *N Engl J Med* 1991;325:1196–204

3. Vane JR, Änggård EE, Botting RM. Regulatory functions of the vascular endothelium. *N Engl J Med* 1990;323:27–36

4. Steinleitner A, Stanczyk FZ, Levin JH, *et al.* Decreased *in vitro* production of 6-keto-prostaglandin $F_{1\alpha}$ by uterine arteries from postmenopausal women. *Am J Obstet Gynecol* 1989;161:1677–81

5. Mikkola T, Turunen P, Avela K, *et al.* 17β-Estradiol stimulates prostacyclin, but not endothelin-1, production in human vascular endothelial cells. *J Clin Endocrinol Metab* 1995;80:1832–6

6. Muck AO, Seeger H, Korte K, *et al.* Natural and synthetic estrogens and prostacyclin production in human endothelial cells from umbilical cord and leg veins. *Prostaglandins* 1993;45:517–25

7. Corvazier E, Dupuy E, Dosne AM, *et al.* Minimal effect of estrogens on endothelial cell growth and production of prostacyclin. *Thrombosis Res* 1984;34:303–10

8. Mikkola T, Ranta V, Orpana A, *et al.* Effect of physiological concentrations of estradiol on PGI_2

and NO in endothelial cells. *Maturitas* 1996; 25:141–7

9. Kibira S, Dudek R, Narayan KS, *et al.* Release of prostacyclin, endothelium-derived relaxing factor and endothelin by freshly harvested cells attached to microcarrier beads. *Mol Cell Biochem* 1991;108:75–84

10. Orpana A, Avela K, Ranta V, *et al.* The calcium-dependent nitric oxide pro-duction of human vascular endothelial cells in preeclampsia. *Am J Obstet Gynecol* 1996;174:1056–60

11. Orpana A, Ranta V, Mikkola T, *et al.* Inducible nitric oxide and prostacyclin productions are differently controlled by extracellular matrix and cell density in human vascular endothelial cells. *J Cell Biochem* 1997;64:538–46

12. Ylikorkala O, Orpana A, Puolakka J, *et al.* Postmenopausal hormonal replace-ment decreases plasma levels of endothelin-1. *J Clin Endocrinol Metab* 1995;80:3384–7

13. Hayashi T, Yamada K, Esaki T, *et al.* Estrogen increases endothelial nitric oxide by a receptor mediated system. *Biochem Biophys Res Commun* 1995;214:847–55

14. Hishikawa K, Nakaki T, Marumo T, *et al.* Up-regulation of nitric oxide synthase by estradiol in human aortic endothelial cells. *FEBS Lett* 1995;360:291–3

15. Schray-Utz B, Zeiher AM, Busse R. Expression of constitutive NO synthase in cultured endothelial

cells is enhanced by 17β-estradiol. *Circulation* 1993;88:I-80

16. Sayegh HS, Ohara Y, Navas JP, *et al.* Endothelial nitric oxide synthase regulation by estrogens. *Circulation* 1993;88:I-80

17. Gilligan DM, Badar DM, Panza JA, *et al.* Acute vascular effects of estrogen in postmenopausal women. *Circulation* 1994;90:786–91

18. Gilligan DM, Badar DM, Panza JA, *et al.* Effects of estrogen replacement therapy on peripheral vasomotor function in postmenopausal women. *Am J Cardiol* 1995;75:264–8

19. Volterrani M, Rosano G, Coats A, *et al.* Estrogen acutely increases peripheral blood flow in postmenopausal women. *Am J Med* 1995;99:119–22

20. Mikkola T, Ristimäki A, Viinikka L, *et al.* Human serum, plasma, and platelets stimulate prostacyclin and endothelin-1 synthesis in human vascular endothelial cells. *Life Sci* 1993;53:283–9

21. Mikkola T, Ranta V, Orpana A, *et al.* Hormone replacement therapy modifies the capacity of plasma and serum to regulate prostacyclin and endothelin-1 production in human vascular endothelial cells. *Fertil Steril* 1996;66:389–93

22. Whitehead M. Progestins and androgens. *Fertil Steril* 1994;62(Suppl. 2):161S–167S

The effect of estrogen on the coronary vasculature $\quad$ 4

P. Collins

HEART DISEASE IN WOMEN

Cardiovascular disease is currently the most common cause of mortality in women and is responsible for the deaths of more women than is cancer, accidents and diabetes combined[1]. Whilst there is no scientific basis for the opinion that cardiovascular disease is a disease restricted to men, there are clearly age-related differences between the two sexes. The incidence of cardiovascular disease in men increases progressively from about the age of 35, while in women a rapid increase is not observed until after the age of 55; by the age of 70 the rates are almost the same.

Cardiovascular diseases are also a major cause of disability in women[1]. Not only do women present with coronary heart disease later in life than men, but they more frequently present with angina and less frequently with sudden death. In 1980, ischemic heart disease was assessed to be disabling in 36% of women aged 55–64, and 55% in women aged 75 and older[2]. The fact that cardiovascular disease is as much a problem of women as of men is not always reflected in treatment patterns. Although women experience chest pain as the main symptom of coronary artery disease more frequently than men, fewer women are referred for major diagnostic or therapeutic tests[3,4]. Angina in women is more difficult to assess, as the diagnostic reliability of tests such as the exercise test is reduced in women; there is a greater chance of having 'ischemic' ECG changes (exercise-induced ST segment depression) in the absence of significant obstructive coronary artery disease. In older women with exertional angina the specificity and sensitivity of the exercise test is increased.

Studies, both in Europe and North America, have shown that men with significant coronary heart disease are more likely than women to undergo revascularization[3–5]. Although there are a number of logical factors that might explain this apparent difference[6], some evidence suggests that, despite the greater incidence of disability associated with cardiovascular disease in women, physicians tend to pursue a less aggressive approach to the management and treatment of coronary disease in women as compared to men[3].

Women have higher complication and mortality rates after myocardial infarction than men[7–9], probably owing to older age and more advanced disease. After thrombolytic therapy for myocardial infarction, women and men have similar morbidity and mortality rates, but women suffer more hemorrhagic stroke[10]. Women undergoing percutaneous transluminal coronary angioplasty tend to have more initial complications and a higher mortality rate than men[11]. This may be explained by a worse risk profile pre-procedure in women compared to men. Clinical success rates were comparable in men and women, as was the 4-year survival rate. Women have a higher mortality rate after coronary artery bypass graft surgery; they are older, more often diabetic and have smaller vessels for grafting[12].

EFFECT OF THE MENOPAUSE

Cardiovascular disease rarely affects women before the menopause, strongly implicating estrogen deficiency in the etiology of the disease. It also suggests that naturally produced estrogens protect women from coronary heart disease before the menopause and that therapeutic estrogens may therefore be expected to do so after it. Support for this hypothesis comes from studies such as the Nurses' Health Study, which showed that the risk of coronary heart disease was more than doubled in women who had bilateral oophorectomy before the menopause, compared with other women of a similar age[13]. A review of population-based case–control, cross-sectional and prospective studies of estrogen therapy (with most using conjugated equine estrogens) and coronary heart disease calculated the overall relative risk associated with estrogen therapy to be reduced by approximately 50%[14].

The first large randomized study of hormone therapy in women with coronary heart disease was recently published[15]. It demonstrated that 0.625 mg of conjugated equine estrogens plus 2.5 mg of medroxy-progesterone acetate in a continuous combined regimen did not have a benefit on the combined end-point of coronary heart disease death and myocardial infarction in women with coronary heart disease. The study suggested an early adverse effect after starting therapy with this combination of hormone therapy. The early adverse effect was small and in the long term there appeared to be a protective effect. There are a number of possible explanations for these results. There are a number of reports that clearly show a detrimental effect of medroxyprogesterone acetate on the beneficial effects of conjugated equine estrogens with regard to atheroma development[16,17] and vascular reactivity[18,19]. There are also studies showing that progesterone does not appear to have this inhibitory effect either on atheroma development[20,21] or vascular reactivity in animal models[19,22] or on vascular reactivity[23] and exercise-induced myocardial ischemia in humans[24].

These results indicate the need for further research into the issue of hormone therapy in older women who have documented coronary heart disease or who are at increased risk of having vascular disease. Conjugated

equine estrogens and medroxyprogesterone acetate at these doses should be avoided. Further randomized studies, investigating different estrogens, progestins, doses, and routes of administration, in different patient populations will be required before definitive conclusions can be made with regard to hormone therapy and cardioprotection.

EFFECT OF ESTROGEN ON THE VESSEL WALL

Endothelium-independent direct vascular smooth muscle relaxation

17β-Estradiol has direct vascular smooth muscle, endothelium-independent relaxing properties on coronary and cerebral blood vessels. In isolated rabbit coronary arteries, Jiang and colleagues[25] demonstrated direct vascular smooth muscle relaxation by pharmacological concentrations of 17β-estradiol. Inhibitors of endothelium-derived relaxing factor (EDRF) did not affect 17β-estradiol-induced relaxation in endothelium-intact coronary arteries.

There are some important differences between isolated human and animal coronary arteries with regard to the relaxation responses to estrogen[26,27]. Atherosclerosis-free male and female human epicardial coronary arteries from patients undergoing heart, or combined heart and lung, transplantation were studied[27]. At physiological concentrations, 17β-estradiol induced significant relaxation in coronary arteries pre-contracted with the thromboxane A_2 analog U46619. Relaxation was significantly greater in coronary arteries from female compared to male patients. No differences were observed between arteries with or without endothelium, nor after nitric oxide synthase or cyclo-oxygenase inhibition. These results indicate that 17β-estradiol induces human coronary artery relaxation by an endothelium-independent mechanism *in vitro*. The gender of the patients significantly affected the sensitivity of the coronary arterial rings to estrogen. The mechanism of this difference remains to be determined. These data from humans are in contrast to data from animal coronary arteries where the relaxation response to estrogen is not gender-dependent and occurs at pharmacological concentrations.

Estrogen and calcium antagonism

Calcium antagonistic properties of estrogen have been suggested from data obtained from uterine arteries[28,29]. 17β-Estradiol-induced inhibition of potential-sensitive calcium channel activation has been demonstrated in animal coronary arteries[25]. 17β-Estradiol induced relaxation of contraction evoked by prostaglandin $(PG)F_{2\alpha}$, an agonist of receptor-operated calcium channels, indicating that 17β-estradiol has similar relaxing effects on contraction induced by activation of both receptor-operated and potential-operated calcium channels. Furthermore, incubation with 17β-estradiol shifted calcium concentration-dependent contraction curves to the right in high potassium-depolarization medium in both coronary arteries and aorta. These findings suggest that 17β-estradiol may have a calcium antagonistic property in these arterial preparations. Confirmation of a calcium antagonistic property of estrogen was provided by experiments on isolated animal cardiac myocytes[30]. The effect of 17β-estradiol on cardiac cell contraction, inward calcium current and intracellular free calcium was investigated using a photodiode array, voltage-clamp and Fura-2 fluorescence techniques, respectively. 17β-Estradiol had a negative inotropic effect on single ventricular myocytes by inhibiting inward calcium current and so reducing intracellular free calcium. This calcium antagonistic property could be one of the mechanisms of 17β-estradiol-induced endothelium-independent relaxation in isolated rabbit and human coronary arterial preparations. Estrogen can relax epicardial coronary arteries by inhibiting calcium influx without changing the calcium sensitivity of contractile elements[31]. This report further reinforces the possibility that a long-term calcium-antagonist

mechanism of estrogen may play a role in its anti-atherosclerotic effect[32].

It has been hypothesized that some of the cardiovascular benefit of estrogen replacement therapy may be due to a calcium antagonist effect of estrogen[32]. In a long-term study of estrogen in atherosclerotic, ovariectomized cynomolgus monkeys, a decrease in coronary atheroma was reported compared to the non-treated animals[33]. Long-term calcium antagonist treatment is known to decrease the progression of atheroma when given to patients with established coronary heart disease[34,35], therefore estrogen may be cardioprotective via a beneficial effect on atheroma progression *in vivo* owing to its calcium antagonistic properties. This hypothesis remains to be proven.

As well as effects on calcium channels, estrogen affects large conductance chloride channels by a direct membrane effect[36]. These channels, in cultured fibroblasts, were inhibited by exposure to extracellular, but not intracellular anti-estrogen, and this effect could be prevented by extracellular 17β-estradiol but not intracellular 17β-estradiol or extracellular 17α-estradiol. This demonstrates another regulatory role for ovarian steroids, affecting plasma ion channels via membrane binding sites distinct from the classical estrogen receptor and subsequent activation of intracellular second-messenger pathway(s).

OTHER VASCULAR EFFECTS OF ESTROGEN

Endothelin-1

Estrogen inhibits the constrictor responses to endothelin-1 in rabbit coronary arteries[37]. Plasma endothelin-1 levels increase following acetylcholine infusion in pigs with coronary atheroma[38] and, although this has not yet been confirmed in humans, it may suggest that the reversal of the constrictor effect of acetylcholine in human atherosclerotic coronary arteries *in vivo* by estrogen[39–41] may be partially explained by estrogen-induced inhibition of endothelin-1-induced contraction.

Estrogen can inhibit responses to vascular constrictor factors such as noradrenaline (norepinephrine), phenylephrine and 5-hydroxytryptamine and the production of factors such as angiotensin II[37,42–45]. Some of these mechanisms may play a role in the long-term vascular protection that is conferred by estrogen replacement therapy.

Renin–angiotensin system

Estrogen inhibits angiotensin II-induced vascular constrictor effects both *in vitro* and *in vivo*, suggesting an inhibitory effect on the renin–angiotensin system. It has been suggested that estrogen is an angiotensin converting enzyme (ACE) inhibitor. By measuring ACE activity and the angiotensin peptides (angiotensin I, angiotensin II and angiotensin (1–7)) in cynomolgus monkeys, it was shown that 30 months of Premarin® treatment decreased ACE activity whereas a combination of Premarin plus medroxyprogesterone acetate increased ACE activity[44]. A study in postmenopausal women confirms an effect of hormone therapy on ACE activity in humans[45]. After 6 months of estrogen/progestogen therapy, serum ACE activity was significantly reduced compared to non-treated controls. Gonadal steroids could therefore confer a beneficial effect on coronary heart disease risk by their effect on ACE.

Prostacyclin

Prostacyclin (PGI2) is a prostaglandin produced by the endothelial cells and its synthesis is coupled to EDRF release[46]. It can induce vasodilatation and inhibition of platelet activation. Estrogen can up-regulate the production of prostacyclin[47]. Chang and co-workers[48] demonstrated an enhancement of basal levels of prostacyclin secretion in rat aortic smooth muscle cells exposed to estradiol. This was thought to be mediated via an increase in transcription of genes for the enzymes prostacyclin synthetase and prostaglandin cyclo-oxygenase. The evidence is scant, however, and has yet to be demonstrated in human tissue, but there is an indication that estrogen may affect coagulation and vasorelaxation by its effects on prostacyclin, since nitric oxide and prostacyclin have been shown favorably to modulate monocyte–vascular wall interactions[49].

Endothelium-dependent mechanisms: nitric oxide

The endothelium is a monolayer of cells which lines the intimal surface of the entire circulatory system and plays an important role in the modulation of vascular tone by the synthesis and secretion of a large array of substances. Endothelium-derived relaxing factor, now known to be nitric oxide[50,51], is one of these substances.

Nitric oxide causes vasorelaxation in endothelium-intact coronary arteries and is a product of the conversion of L-arginine by nitric oxide synthases to nitric oxide and citrulline. Nitric oxide synthase can be divided into two functional groups based on their calcium sensitivity. Estrogen can enhance the amount of available intracellular nitric oxide synthase by inducing calcium-dependent nitric oxide synthase[52]. There is an increased basal release of nitric oxide from female rabbit endothelium-intact aortic rings compared with that from males[53]. Estrogen-induced increases in blood flow in the uterine artery *in vivo* can be antagonized by nitric oxide synthase inhibition[54]. Nitric oxide has also been observed to slow the development of atheroma by inhibiting smooth cell proliferation while stimulating proliferation of endothelial cells[55]. Estrogen is a potent antioxidant of lipids[56], and oxidized lipids inhibit nitric oxide[57]. Estrogen may therefore be vasculoprotective via enhanced nitric oxide production and/or by reducing nitric oxide breakdown. The time course for this potential anti-atherogenic effect is unknown and may be relevant only with long-term estrogen treatment.

A study in humans demonstrated variation in expired nitric oxide production with cyclical hormone changes in premenopausal women, with nitric oxide levels peaking at the middle of the menstrual cycle[58], suggesting an influence of gonadal hormones on the synthesis and release of nitric oxide in humans.

There is a growing body of evidence from different animal models that estrogen can enhance nitric oxide production from the vascular endothelium. The precise mechanism(s) involved remain to be fully identified.

Estrogen and nitric oxide synthase

Estrogen can stimulate nitric oxide synthase in cultured bovine and human umbilical endothelial cells, this effect is estrogen receptor dependent[59]. Short exposure to estrogen stimulates basal nitric oxide synthase in cultured human umbilical vein endothelial cultured monolayers within 60 mins, this effect is independent of cytosolic calcium mobilization[60]. Sex hormones have effects on calcium-dependent nitric oxide production and protein levels of nitric oxide synthase in cultured human aortic endothelial cells. Endothelial nitric oxide stimulation was shown to occur at physiological concentrations of 17β-estradiol. The increase in nitric oxide synthase activity was partially inhibited by tamoxifen, suggesting that the effect on the nitric oxide synthase was via the classical receptor. Testosterone had no effect on nitric oxide synthase[61]. These data confirm that human endothelial nitric oxide synthase can be regulated by estrogens *in vitro*.

An *in vivo* study in guinea pigs examined the effects of estrogen on nitric oxide synthase activity in heart, kidney and skeletal muscle. Estradiol increased nitric oxide production in female guinea pigs after 5 days' treatment. However, this occurred in males only after 10 days of estrogen exposure[52]. It was suggested that the number or availability of estrogen receptors in male tissues is initially too low, requiring a period of estrogen priming.

The sex hormone status of the animal may be important in determining whether nitric oxide plays a role in the estrogen-induced coronary and basilar artery relaxation[62,63]. Female rabbits that were estrogen-treated and then had estrogen acutely withdrawn (mimicking a perimenopausal state) demonstrated an increased sensitivity to the relaxing effect of 17β-estradiol, which was found to be endothelium- and nitric oxide-dependent. Estrogen-induced, endothelium-dependent relaxation of coronary arteries may therefore, in some species, depend on the sex hormone status of the animal.

Estrogen receptor

Estrogen receptor-dependent mechanisms are involved in the response of blood vessels of the reproductive system to gonadal hormones, and estrogen receptors are found in a number of other tissues including the heart and liver[64,65]. Recent data suggest that some of the acute effects of estrogen in other circulations may be independent of the classical estrogen receptor. Receptor-dependent mechanisms may be involved in chronic vascular effects, but there are no data that prove this hypothesis. There are conflicting data on the presence of estrogen receptors in human female coronary arteries. They have been demonstrated in normal coronary arteries, however there is variable expression in atherosclerotic coronary arteries from premenopausal women[66]. Others have found no evidence for estrogen receptors in normal coronary arteries, using a different antibody technique[67]. Studies using specific monoclonal antibodies and nuclear probes have confirmed the presence of a classical estrogen receptor in cultured human umbilical, aortic and coronary artery endothelial cells[68,69], suggesting that the cardioprotective effect of estrogen may, at least in part, be due to effects on endothelial cell function via the estrogen receptor. A novel estrogen receptor has recently been cloned in rat prostate, and is called estrogen-receptor-beta, or ER-β[70]. This receptor was also found in the ovary and had high affinity to 17β-estradiol. At present, no such receptor has been identified in human tissue, but this finding raises the possibility of vascular-specific estrogen receptors that may be involved in the modulation of vascular responses to estrogen.

IN VIVO CORONARY VASCULAR RESPONSES TO ESTROGEN

Direct vascular smooth muscle effects

Estrogen induces dilatation of conductance and resistance coronary arteries, albeit at supraphysiological concentrations (> 0.1 μmol/l), in dogs when administered acutely into the coronary circulation[71]. By removing the endothelium and using inhibitors of adenosine triphosphate-sensitive potassium and calcium channels, it was shown that this effect is endothelium-independent and is partially mediated by effects on adenosine triphosphate-sensitive potassium and/or calcium channels. Experiments using a classic intracellular estrogen receptor antagonist showed that the receptor is not involved in the response.

Indirect endothelium-dependent effects

In ovariectomized animals, long-term (2 years)[72] estrogen replacement therapy reverses acetylcholine-induced constriction in atherosclerotic coronary arteries, and a similar effect is produced with a 20-min intravenous infusion of ethinyl estradiol[73]. These animal data have been reproduced in postmenopausal women with coronary atherosclerosis. Estrogen attenuates[39] or abolishes[40,41] acetylcholine-induced vasoconstriction when administered acutely (15–20 min after bolus or continuous intracoronary infusion) in these women, resulting in increased coronary diameter and flow. This response of the coronary arteries to acetylcholine after exposure to 17β-estradiol appears to be gender dependent[41]. A 20-min exposure to 17β-estradiol modulated acetylcholine-induced responses of female but not male atherosclerotic coronary arteries *in vivo*. Current, chronic, physiological estrogen replacement has also been shown to influence endothelium-dependent and -independent coronary responsiveness to acetylcholine[74]. Estrogen replacement therapy was associated with an attenuation or reversal of the coronary vasoconstrictor response to acetylcholine in postmenopausal women. This suggests a possible normalization of an endothelium-dependent mechanism in diseased coronary vessels, in agreement with the effect of acutely administered estrogen. Such an effect could contribute to an estrogen-induced reduction in cardiovascular events associated with estrogen therapy.

RELEVANCE OF VASCULAR EFFECTS OF ESTROGEN TO POTENTIAL THERAPEUTIC OPTION FOR CARDIOVASCULAR DISEASE

Myocardial ischemia

Estrogen-induced reduction in vascular resistance and increases in coronary flow may have clinical implications with regard to exercise-induced myocardial ischemia, where coronary stenoses may become flow limiting. Rosano and colleagues[75] demonstrated a beneficial effect of acute administration of sublingual 17β-estradiol versus placebo on signs of exercise-induced myocardial ischemia on the electrocardiogram (time to 1 mm ST-segment depression) and exercise tolerance in postmenopausal women. Patients with low plasma 17β-estradiol levels generally had a greater response to 17β-estradiol. Plasma levels achieved in this study were in the order of 2500 pmol/l, which is above the peak level found at mid-cycle (mid-cycle level approximately 1800 pmol/l) and about one-third of the level found in pregnancy. This effect may be due to a direct relaxing effect on the coronary arteries[27], peripheral vasodilatation[76], or a combination of the two. Further confirmation of a beneficial effect of acutely administered conjugated estrogen on myocardial ischemia in postmenopausal women with coronary heart disease has been provided by Alpaslan *et al*.[77]. They investigated the effect of intravenous estrogen on myocardial function using dobutamine stress echocardiography, showing an improvement in ischemic end points after estrogen when compared to placebo infusion. An anti-ischemic effect of acute sublingual estrogen in postmenopausal women has been demonstrated at physiological plasma estrogen levels using coronary sinus pH measurements during atrial pacing-induced myocardial ischemia[78].

The question of longer-term treatment has recently been addressed. Treatment for 4 and 8 weeks with transdermal 17β-estradiol improves exercise time to myocardial ischemia in postmenopausal women with documented coronary heart disease[79]. In this study the plasma levels of estrogen were within the expected range for postmenopausal estrogen treatment.

Further studies will be required to assess the efficacy of estrogen therapy in the treatment of angina in the presence of coronary artery disease.

Cardiological syndrome X

Angina pectoris is usually caused by obstructive atheromatous coronary artery disease; however, angiographically smooth coronary arteries are found in approximately 20% of patients who undergo coronary angiography[80] and the majority of these patients are women. The triad of angina pectoris, a positive exercise test and angiographically smooth coronary arteries is commonly referred to as syndrome X, a term first used by Kemp and colleagues in 1973[81]. The pathophysiology of the troublesome chest pain in syndrome X is poorly understood, and there are many suggested mechanisms[82-84]. Although syndrome X is likely to be a heterogeneous condition, reduced coronary flow reserve induced by dipyridamole has been reported in many patients with this diagnosis[83,85]. Most of the women with syndrome X are postmenopausal[86] and a

recent study which investigated the clinical and gynecological features of female patients with syndrome X found that ovarian hormone deficiency played a role in unmasking the syndrome in female patients[87]. Estrogen therapy may be helpful in the treatment of this condition by decreasing the occurrence of chest pain[88]. There was no effect on exercise tolerance, which may be related to the fact that only a small number of patients with syndrome X suffer true myocardial ischemia.

Supraventricular tachycardia

A recent study in healthy premenopausal women showed cyclical variation in the occurrence of paroxysmal supraventricular tachycardia (SVT) with the menstrual cycle, and a relationship between ovarian hormones and paroxysmal SVT[89]. An increased incidence of SVT was found during the luteal phase of the menstrual cycle, possibly linked to increased sympathetic activity. This could be a result of decreased estrogen levels and/or increased progesterone levels. Electrophysiological effects of estrogen on the heart are relatively unexplored.

CONCLUSIONS

Heart disease is as common in women as in men; however, it occurs in women later in life. The menopause, and its associated estrogen deficiency, appear to be risk factors for the development of cardiovascular disease in women, and postmenopausal estrogen therapy has been shown to decrease this risk.

Estrogen decreases vascular tone by a number of different mechanisms, including endothelium-derived nitric oxide and prostanoids, ion channel modulation, inhibition of constrictor factors and others. Advantageous effects on acute and chronic blood flow by estrogen may also involve these mechanisms, and they may at least partially account for the beneficial effects of estrogen on atherogenesis.

Whether hormone therapy is, or is not cardio-protective in the long term, particularly in women with established coronary heart disease, will require more randomized clinical trials. There is a wealth of epidemiological evidence to suggest that it is. It is up to clinical scientists to further investigate this question in order to be able to give definitive answers to postmenopausal women who are about to start, or who are already taking hormone therapy. Further randomized trials will be required to confirm or refute this notion.

References

1. Eaker E, Chesebro JH, Sacks FM, *et al.* Cardiovascular disease in women. *Circulation* 1993;88:1999–2009
2. Pinsky JL, Jette AM, Branch LG, *et al.* The Framingham Disability Study: relationship of various coronary heart disease manifestations to disability in older persons living in the community. *Am J Public Health* 1990;80:1363–7
3. Steingart RM, Packer M, Hamm P, *et al.* Sex differences in the management of coronary artery disease. Survival and ventricular enlargement investigators. *N Engl J Med* 1991;325:226–30
4. Ayanian JZ, Epstein AM. Differences in the use of procedures between men and women hospitalised for coronary heart disease. *N Engl J Med* 1991;325:221–5
5. Pettigrew M, McKee M, Jones J. Coronary artery surgery: are women discriminated against? *Br Med J* 1993;306:1164–6
6. Mark DB, Shaw LK, DeLong ER, *et al.* Absence of sex bias in the referral of patients for cardiac catheterization. *Circulation* 1994;330:1101–6
7. Gomez-Marin O, Folsom AR, Kottke TE, *et al.* Improvement in long-term survival among patients hospitalized with acute myocardial infarction. *N Engl J Med* 1987;316:1353–9
8. Dittrich H, Gilpin E, Nicod P, *et al.* Acute myocardial infarction in women: influence of gender on mortality and prognostic variables. *Am J Cardiol* 1988;62:1–7
9. Puletti M, Sunseri L, Curione M, *et al.* Acute myocardial infarction: sex related differences in prognosis. *Am Heart J* 1984;108:63–6
10. White HD, Barbash GI, Modan M, *et al.* After correcting for worse baseline characteristics, women treated with thrombolytic therapy for acute myocardial infarction have the same mortality and morbidity as men except for a higher incidence of hemorrhagic stroke. *Circulation* 1993;88:2097–2103
11. Kelsey SF, James M, Holubkov AL, *et al.* Results of percutaneous transluminal coronary angioplasty in women. *Circulation* 1993;87:720–27
12. O'Connor GT, Morton JR, Diehl MJ, *et al.* Differences between men and women in hospital mortality associated with coronary artery bypass graft surgery. *Circulation* 1993;88:2104–10
13. Colditz GA, Willett WC, Stampfer MJ, *et al.* Menopause and the risk of coronary heart disease in women. *N Engl J Med* 1987;316:1105–10
14. Stampfer MJ, Colditz GA. Estrogen replacement therapy and coronary heart disease: a quantitative assessment of the epidemiologic evidence. *Preventive Med* 1991;20:47–63
15. Hulley S, Grady D, Bush T, *et al.* Randomized trial of estrogen plus progestin for secondary prevention of coronary heart disease in postmenopausal women. Heart and Estrogen/progestin Replacement Study (HERS) Research Group. *J Am Med Assoc* 1998;280:605–13
16. Adams MR, Register TC, Golden DL, *et al.* Medroxyprogesterone acetate antagonizes inhibitory effects of conjugated equine estrogens on coronary artery atherosclerosis. *Arterioscler Thromb Vasc Biol* 1997;17:217–21
17. Levine RL, Chen SJ, Durand J, *et al.* Medroxyprogesterone attenuates estrogen-mediated inhibition of neointima formation after balloon injury of the rat carotid artery. *Circulation* 1996;94:2221–27
18. Williams JK, Honore EK, Washburn SA, *et al.* Effects of hormone replacement therapy on reactivity of atherosclerotic coronary arteries in cynomolgus monkeys. *J Am Coll Cardiol* 1994;24:1757–61
19. Miyagawa K, Rosch J, Stanczyk F, *et al.* Medroxyprogesterone interferes with ovarian steroid protection against coronary vasospasm. *Nature Med* 1997;3:324–7
20. Adams MR, Kaplan JR, Manuck SB, *et al.* Inhibition of coronary artery atherosclerosis by 17-beta estradiol in ovariectomized monkeys. Lack of an effect on added progesterone. *Arteriosclerosis* 1995;10:1051–7
21. Register TC, Adams MR, Golden DL, *et al.* Conjugated equine estrogens alone, but not in combination with medroxyprogesterone acetate, inhibit aortic connective tissue remodeling after

plasma lipid lowering in female monkeys. *Arterioscler Thromb Vasc Biol* 1998;18:1164–71

22. Jiang C, Sarrel PM, Lindsay DC, *et al.* Progesterone induces endothelium-independent relaxation of rabbit coronary artery in vitro. *Eur J Pharmacol* 1992;211:163–7

23. Gerhard M, Walsh BW, Tawakol A, *et al.* Estradiol therapy combined with progesterone and endothelium-dependent vasodilation in postmenopausal women. *Circulation* 1998;98:1158–63

24. Rosano GMC, Chierchia SL, Morgagni GL, *et al.* Effect of the association of different progestogens to estradiol 17β therapy upon effort-induced myocardial ischemia in female patients with coronary artery disease. *J Am Coll Cardiol* 1997;29:344(Abstract)

25. Jiang C, Sarrel PM, Lindsay DC, *et al.* Endothelium-independent relaxation of rabbit coronary artery by 17β-oestradiol *in vitro*. *Br J Pharmacol* 1991;104:1033–7

26. Mügge A, Riedel M, Barton M, *et al.* Endothelium independent relaxation of human coronary arteries by 17beta-oestradiol *in vitro*. *Cardiovasc Res* 1993;27:1939–42

27. Chester AH, Jiang C, Borland JA, *et al.* Estrogen relaxes human epicardial coronary arteries through non-endothel-ium-dependent mechanisms. *Cor Art Dis* 1995;6:417–22

28. Stice SL, Ford SP, Rosazza JP, *et al.* Role of 4-hydroxylated estradiol in reducing Ca^{2+} uptake of uterine arterial smooth muscle cells through potential-sensitive channels. *Biol Reprod* 1987;36:361–8

29. Stice SL, Ford SP, Rosazza JP, *et al.* Interaction of 4-hydroxylated estradiol and potential-sensitive Ca^{2+} channels in altering uterine blood flow during the estrous cycle and early pregnancy in gilts. *Biol Reprod* 1987;36:369–75

30. Jiang C, Poole-Wilson PA, Sarrel PM, *et al.* Effect of 17β-oestradiol on contraction, Ca^{2+} current and intracellular free Ca^{2+} in guinea-pig isolated cardiac myocytes. *Br J Pharmacol* 1992;106:739–45

31. Han SZ, Karaki H, Ouchi Y, *et al.* 17β-Estradiol inhibits Ca^{2+} influx and Ca^{2+} release induced by thromboxane A2 in porcine coronary artery. *Circulation* 1995;91:2619–26

32. Collins P, Rosano GMC, Jiang C, *et al.* Hypothesis: cardiovascular protection by oestrogen – a calcium antagonist effect? *Lancet* 1993;341:1264–5

33. Adams MR, Kaplan JR, Manuck SB, *et al.* Inhibition of coronary artery atherosclerosis by 17-beta estradiol in ovariectomized monkeys. Lack of an effect of added progesterone. *Arteriosclerosis* 1990;10:1051–7

34. Lichtlen PR, Hugenholtz PG, Rafflenbeul W, *et al.* Retardation of angiographic progression of coronary artery disease by nifedipine. *Lancet* 1990;335:1109–13

35. Waters D, Lesperance J, Francetich M, *et al.* A controlled clinical trial to assess the effect of a calcium channel blocker on the progression of coronary atherosclerosis. *Circulation* 1990;82:1940–53

36. Hardy SP, Valverde MA. Novel plasma membrane action of estrogen and antiestrogens revealed by their regulation of a large conductance chloride channel. *FASEB J* 1994;8:760–65

37. Jiang C, Sarrel PM, Poole-Wilson PA, *et al.* Acute effect of 17β-estradiol on rabbit coronary artery contractile responses to endothelin-1. *Am J Physiol* 1992;263:H271–H275

38. Lerman A, Webster MWI, Chesebro JH, *et al.* Circulating and tissue endothelin immuno-reactivity in hypercholesterolemic pigs. *Circulation* 1993;88:2923–8

39. Reis SE, Gloth ST, Blumenthal RS, *et al.* Ethinyl estradiol acutely attenuates abnormal coronary vasomotor responses to acetylcholine in post-menopausal women. *Circulation* 1994;89:52–60

40. Gilligan DM, Quyyumi AA, Cannon RO III. Effects of physiological levels of estrogen on coronary vasomotor function in postmenopausal women. *Circulation* 1994;89:2545–51

41. Collins P, Rosano GMC, Sarrel PM, *et al.* Estradiol-17β attenuates acetylcholine-induced coronary arterial con-striction in women but not men with coronary heart disease. *Circulation* 1995;92:24–30

42. Cheng DY, Gruetter CA. Chronic estrogen alters contractile responsiveness to angiotensin II and norepinephrine in female rat aorta. *Eur J Pharmacol* 1992;215:171–6

43. Magness RR, Parker CR Jr, Rosenfeld CR. Systemic and uterine responses to chronic infusion of estradiol-17 beta. *Am J Physiol* 1993;265:E690–E698

44. Brosnihan KB, Weedle D, Anthony MS, *et al.* Does chronic estrogen act as a converting enzyme inhibitor in postmenopausal cyno-molgous monkeys? *Am J Hypertens* 1995;8:107A (Abstract)

45. Proudler AJ, Hasib Ahmed AI, Crook D, *et al.* Hormone replacement therapy and serum angioten-sin-converting-enzyme activity in postmenopausal women. *Lancet* 1995;346:89–90

46. Botting R, Vane JR. The receipt and dispatch of chemical messengers by endothelial cells. In Schrör K, Sinzinger H, eds. *Prostaglandins in Clinical Research: Cardiovascular System.* New York: Alan R Liss, 1989:1–11

47. Mendelsohn ME, Karas RH. Estrogen and the blood vessel wall. *Curr Opin Cardiol* 1994;9:619–26

48. Chang WC, Nakao J, Orimo H, *et al.* Stimulation of prostacyclin biosynthetic activity by estradiol

in rat aortic smooth muscle cells in culture. *Biochim Biophys Acta* 1980;619:107–18

49. Bath PM, Hassall DG, Gladwin AM, *et al.* Nitric oxide and prostacyclin. Divergence of inhibitory effects on monocyte chemotaxis and adhesion to endothelium *in vitro. Arterioscler Thromb* 1991;11:254–60

50. Palmer RM, Ferrige AG, Moncada S. Nitric oxide release accounts for the biological activity of endothelium-derived relaxing factor. *Nature (London)* 1987;327:524–6

51. Myers PR, Guerra RJ, Harrison DG. Release of NO and EDRF from cultured bovine aortic endothelial cells. *Am J Physiol* 1989;256:H1030–H1037

52. Weiner CP, Lizasoain I, Baylis SA, *et al.* Induction of calcium-dependent nitric oxide synthases by sex hormones. *Proc Natl Acad Sci USA* 1994;91:5212–16

53. Hayashi T, Fukuto JM, Ignarro LJ, *et al.* Basal release of nitric oxide from aortic rings is greater in female rabbits than in male rabbits: implications for atherosclerosis. *Proc Natl Acad Sci USA* 1992;89:11259–63

54. Van Buren G, Yang D, Clark KE. Estrogen-induced uterine vasodilatation is antagonized by L-nitroarginine methyl ester, an inhibitor of nitric oxide synthesis. *Am J Obstet Gynecol* 1992;16:828–33

55. Dubey RK, Overbeck HW. Culture of rat mesenteric arteriolar smooth muscle cells: effects of platelet-derived growth factor, angiotensin, and nitric oxide on growth. *Cell Tissue Res* 1994;275:133–41

56. Sack MN, Rader DJ, Cannon RO III. Oestrogen and inhibition of oxidation of low-density lipoproteins in postmenopausal women. *Lancet* 1994;343:269–70

57. Simon BC, Cunningham LD, Cohen RA. Oxidized low density lipoproteins cause contraction and inhibit endothelium-dependent relaxation in the pig coronary artery. *J Clin Invest* 1990;86:75–9

58. Kharitonov SA, Logan-Sinclair RB, Busset CM, *et al.* Peak expiratory nitric oxide differences in men and women: relation to the menstrual cycle. *Br Heart J* 1994;72:243–5

59. Hayashi T, Yamada K, Esaki T, *et al.* Estrogen increases endothelial nitric oxide by a receptor-mediated system. *Biochem Biophys Res Commun* 1995;214:847–55

60. Caulin-Glaser T, Garcia-Cardena G, Sarrel P, *et al.* 17 beta-estradiol regulation of human endothelial cell basal nitric oxide release, independent of cytosolic Ca2+ mobilization. *Circ Res* 1997;81:885–92

61. Hishikawa K, Nakaki T, Marumo T, *et al.* Up-regulation of nitric oxide synthase by estradiol in human aortic endothelial cells. *FEBS Lett* 1995;360:291–3

62. Collins P, Shay J, Jiang C, *et al.* Nitric oxide accounts for dose-dependent estrogen-mediated coronary relaxation following acute estrogen withdrawal. *Circulation* 1994;90:1964–8

63. Futo J, Shay J, Holt J, *et al.* Estrogen and progesterone withdrawl increases cerebral vasoreactivity to serotonin in rabbit basilar artery. *Life Sci* 1992;50:1165–72

64. McGill HC Jr. Sex steroid hormone receptors in the cardiovascular system. *Postgrad Med* 1989;64–8

65. Kahn D, Zeng Q, Kajani M, *et al.* The effect of different types of hepatic injury on the estrogen and androgen receptor activity of liver. *J Invest Surg* 1989;2:125–33

66. Losordo DW, Kearney M, Kim EA, *et al.* Variable expression of the estrogen receptor in normal and atherosclerotic coronary arteries of premenopausal women. *Circulation* 1994;89:1501–10

67. Collins P, Sheppard M, Beale CM, *et al.* The classical estrogen receptor is not found in human coronary arteries. *Circulation* 1995;92:I-37 (Abstract)

68. Venkov CD, Rankin AB, Vaughan DE. Identification of authentic estrogen receptor in cultured endothelial cells. A potential mechanism for steroid hormone regulation of endothelial function. *Circulation* 1996;94:727–33

69. Kim-Schulze S, McGowan KA, Hubchak SC, *et al.* Expression of an estrogen receptor by human coronary artery and umbilical vein endothelial cells. *Circulation* 1996;94:1402–07

70. Kuiper GG, Enmark E, Pelto-Huikko M, *et al.* Cloning of a novel receptor expressed in rat prostate and ovary. *Proc Natl Acad Sci USA* 1996;93:5925–30

71. Sudhir K, Chou TM, Mullen WL, *et al.* Mechanisms of estrogen-induced vasodilation: *in vivo* studies in canine coronary conductance and resistance arteries. *J Am Coll Cardiol* 1995;26:807–14

72. Williams JK, Adams MR, Klopfenstein HS. Estrogen modulates responses of atherosclerotic coronary arteries. *Circulation* 1990;81:1680–87

73. Williams JK, Adams MR, Herrington DM, *et al.* Short-term administration of estrogen and vascular responses of atherosclerotic coronary arteries. *J Am Coll Cardiol* 1992;20:452–7

74. Herrington DM, Braden GA, Williams JK, *et al.* Endothelial-dependent coronary vasomotor responsiveness in postmenopausal women with and without estrogen replacement therapy. *Am J Cardiol* 1994;73:951–2

75. Rosano GMC, Sarrel PM, Poole-Wilson PA, *et al.* Beneficial effect of oestrogen on exercise-induced myocardial ischaemia in women with coronary artery disease. *Lancet* 1993;342:133–6

76. Volterrani M, Rosano GMC, Coats A, *et al.* Estrogen acutely increases peripheral blood flow

in postmenopausal women. *Am J Med* 1995;99: 119–22

77. Alpaslan M, Shimokawa H, Kuroiwa-Matsumoto M, *et al.* Short-term estrogen administration ameliorates dobutamine-induced myocardial ischemia in postmenopausal women with coronary artery disease. *J Am Coll Cardiol* 1997; 30:1466–71

78. Rosano GMC, Caixeta AM, Chierchia SL, *et al.* Acute anti-ischemic effect of estradiol-17β in postmenopausal women with coronary artery disease. *Circulation* 1997;96:2837–41

79. Webb CM, Rosano GMC, Collins P. Oestrogen improves exercise-induced myocardial ischaemia in women. *Lancet* 1998;351:1556–7

80. Likoff W, Segal BL, Kasparian H. Paradox of normal selective coronary arteriograms in patients considered to have unmistakable coronary heart disease. *N Engl J Med* 1967; 276:1063–6

81. Kemp HG Jr, Vokonas PS, Cohn PF, *et al.* The anginal syndrome associated with normal coronary arteriograms. Report of a six year experience. *Am J Med* 1973;54:735–42

82. Maseri A, Crea F, Kaski JC, *et al.* Mechanisms of angina pectoris in syndrome X. *J Am Coll Cardiol* 1991;17:499–506

83. Cannon RO, Epstein SE. 'Microvascular angina' as a cause of chest pain with angiographically normal coronary arteries. *Am J Cardiol* 1988; 61:1338–43

84. Rosano GMC, Lindsay DC, Poole-Wilson PA. Syndrome X: an hypothesis for cardiac pain without ischaemia. *Cardiologia* 1991;36:885–95

85. Opherk D, Zebe H, Weihe E, *et al.* Reduced coronary dilatory capacity and ultrastructural changes of the myocardium in patients with angina pectoris but normal coronary arteriograms. *Circulation* 1981;63:817–25

86. Kaski JC, Rosano GMC, Collins P, *et al.* Cardiac syndrome X: clinical characteristics and left ventricular function. Long term follow-up study. *J Am Coll Cardiol* 1995;25:807–14

87. Rosano GMC, Collins P, Kaski JC, *et al.* Syndrome X in women is associated with estrogen deficiency. *Eur Heart J* 1995;16:610–14

88. Rosano GMC, Peters NS, Lefroy DC, *et al.* 17-beta-estradiol therapy lessens angina in postmenopausal women with syndrome X. *J Am Coll Cardiol* 1996;28:1500–505

89. Rosano GMC, Leonardo F, Sarrel PM, *et al.* Cyclical variation in paroxysmal supraventricular tachycardia in women. *Lancet* 1996;347:786–8

Impact of physiological estradiol replacement therapy on the production of vascular prostacyclin and of nitric oxide by human vascular endothelial cells: an *in vitro* and *in vivo* study

5

J.M. Foidart

Cardiovascular heart disease is the leading cause of mortality and a major cause of morbidity in postmenopausal women. The main risk factors are hypertension, smoking, hyperlipidemia, obesity and diabetes[1]. Many studies have established that estrogen replacement therapy (ERT) in postmenopausal women reduces cardiovascular disease, partly by increasing high-density lipoprotein (HDL) and decreasing low-density lipoprotein (LDL), and by favourably influencing the prostacyclin/thromboxane balance[2]. Estrogens also prevent cholesterol and oxidized LDL particles from accumulating in the arterial wall. They also enhance the production of nitric oxide (NO) by inducing NO synthase expression in endothelial cells. We have previously shown that physiological levels of estrone and estradiol double the production of NO by human vascular endothelial cells *in vitro* and increase the urinary levels of NO_2 and NO_3 by 15%. Endogenous or exogenous estrogens increase coronary blood flow and improve walking distance in angina patients. They decrease the arterial resistance and modify the Doppler velocity waves in uterine and carotid arteries. When administered transdermally, estrogens do not induce their hepatic first-pass effect. There are thus minimal or no changes in the renin–angiotensin–aldosterone system nor in the hepatic synthesis of procoagulant factors. This type of replacement therapy with estradiol should therefore be more often prescribed to women with atherogenic hyperlipidemia, arterial hypertension or ischemic coronary disease.

ERT has not been associated with a rise in blood pressure (BP) in postmenopausal, normotensive women[3]. Peck and co-workers[4] reported, in 31 hypertensive women (23 receiving antihypertensive treatment), a rise in systolic BP in 14 patients, no change in one patient and a decrease in BP in 16 patients receiving various hormone replacement therapy (HRT) regimens. Diastolic BP went up in 11 women, remained unchanged in one woman and fell in 19 women. They concluded that HRT induced no systemically important pressor effect and was safe in hypertensive women. Luotola[5], in a cross-over study versus placebo, showed that the administration of 2 mg and 4 mg per os estradiol lowered BP in normotensive and even in hypertensive subjects.

Synthetic estrogen (namely ethinyl estradiol) used in oral contraception might overstimulate the hepatic production of the renin substrate and angiotensinogen with an increased risk of hypertension, vasoconstriction and platelet aggregation. Conjugated equine estrogens can also, to some extent, exhibit the same stimulatory hepatic effects and their use might also, but more exceptionally, lead to clinically relevant events such as hypertension. Non-orally administered estradiol has minimal or no hepatic impact and this might result in the absence of a negative impact on cardio-vascular disease or may even exert a protective effect. Previous studies have shown that progesterone inhibits the effect of mineralocorticoids and has a natriuretic effect; this would lead to an increase in renin secretion, increased formation of angiotensin I and II and a rise in aldosterone secretion. However, in some studies, it has been demonstrated that progestational and natriuretic effects varied among the different progestins and could influence the renin–aldosterone system in different ways. For example the C_{21} compounds, e.g. medroxy-progesterone acetate (MPA), given at low doses, do not stimulate the renin substrate.

The cardioprotective effect of HRT among normotensive postmenopausal women is widely accepted. However, its use remains controversial in postmenopausal women with hypertension. At present, there are only few epidemiological data on changes in BP in hypertensive women receiving HRT. We observed no clinically significant differences in BP (both systolic and diastolic) among 150 hypertensive postmenopausal users of Estra-derm TTS 50 + MPA between measurements before and during treatment. Most studies have found no change or even a reduction in BP with estrogen use. We may conclude from our study that ERT by transdermal estradiol administration to hypertensive women with well-controlled hypertension is safe and might even be beneficial, since this treatment produces a significant reduction in other coronary risks factors. Such treatments would ideally involve co-operation between the cardiologist, the gynecologist and the general practitioner. In conclusion, Estraderm TTS 50 continuously and MPA 10 mg/day during the first 12 days of each month can be used safely as HRT in postmenopausal women with therapeutically controlled hypertension.

References

1. Radwanska E. The role of reproductive hormones in vascular disease and hypertension. *Steroids* 1993;58:605–10

2. Foidart JM, Dombrowicz N, de Lignières B. Urinary excretion of prostacyclin and thromboxane metabolites in postmenopausal women treated with percutaneous estradiol (Oestrogel®) or conjugated estrogens (Premarin®). In Dusitsin N, Notelovitz M, eds. *Physiological Hormone Replacement Therapy.* Carnforth, UK: Parthenon Publishing, 1991:99–107

3. Wren GB, Routledge AD. The effect of type and dose of oestrogen on the blood pressure of post-menopausal women. *Maturitas* 1983;5:135

4. Peck K, Perry IJ, Lusesly DM, *et al.* Effect of hormone replacement therapy on blood pressure in hypertension. *J Hypertens* 1991;II:1087

5. Luotola H. Blood pressure and haemodynamics in postmenopausal women during estradiol-17-beta substitution. *Ann Clin Rev* 1983;15:1

Alterations in cardiac hemodynamics associated with menopause and HRT

6

A. Pines

HORMONE DEFICIENCY AND THE HEART

M-mode echocardiographic examinations of healthy postmenopausal women showed that their left ventricle (LV) is relatively thicker than that of premenopausal women of the same age[1]. Moreover, Doppler echocardiographic studies disclosed an inverse correlation between the time-lapse since menopause and the aortic blood flow velocity and acceleration, indicating a relatively less effective LV function[2]. These findings may represent very early signs of LV dysfunction, which could be related to the increase in the incidence of coronary artery disease known to occur after menopause. Similar results were obtained when Doppler echocardiography was performed in cases of chemically induced menopause, namely in young women undergoing fertility treatment with a gonadotropin releasing hormone (GnRH) agonist: blood flow velocity and acceleration decreased when estrogen levels fell to menopausal values as a result of therapy[3].

There have been only limited data on possible pathophysiological mechanisms which could explain this association between cardiac function and menopause. One of these mechanisms is probably related to endothelial function, which declines with age. In women, this decline is delayed until the beginning of the menopausal transition, but it starts earlier in men, i.e. at the age of 40[4]. Many non-reproductive-system organs (including the heart and vessels) include physiologically active estrogen receptors which are able to regulate gene expression. Among such target genes are those of angiotensin converting enzyme (ACE), nitric oxide synthase and prostaglandin cyclooxygenase, which are important factors in the regulation of myocardial blood flow. Estrogen deficiency alters the activity and probably the density of estrogen receptors. Estrogen status also determines, to some extent, the ratio of V1/V3 myosin isoforms[5]. Since the level of the less contractable isoform, the V3 (beta) isomyosin, increases in menopause, the above-mentioned changes in cardiac performance related to menopause could be the end result of such an effect. Furthermore, estrogen status may partially regulate the expression of several proto-oncogenes involved in cardiac hypertrophy, again pointing toward the diversity of mechanisms by which ovarian function, cardiac anatomy and cardiac hemodynamics could be interrelated.

HORMONE REPLACEMENT THERAPY AND THE HEART

If hormone deficiency is associated with less effective LV performance and thickening of the left ventricular walls, then the reverse can be expected when hormone substitution is administered. Indeed, 3 months' hormone therapy in healthy postmenopausal women resulted in an increase in the Doppler parameters of aortic blood flow as compared to pretreatment values, with the effect being maintained for a year[6]. A reduction in LV wall width was observed in healthy women using transdermal estradiol for 1.5 years. In another study, we divided postmenopausal women with mild hypertension into hormone users and non-users, and echocardiographic examinations were performed at baseline and after 6–12 months[7]. We observed a decrease in cardiac size which was the result of both a reduction in heart volume and wall thickness in the hormone users. We also found that they had an increase in aortic blood flow velocity and acceleration. These findings were absent in the non-users. Moreover, hormone users were shown to have a more blunted blood pressure response during dynamic and isometric exercise, as compared to the controls. The smaller increments in blood pressure during exercise could be interpreted as expressing an advantage to hormone users, since it probably indicates a more effective LV function, together with reduced oxygen consumption on exertion.

A minimal period of time is apparently needed in order to detect anatomic and functional changes in the myocardium during hormone substitution. This is probably why most studies on the cardiovascular effects of estrogen allowed more than 2 months of therapy before re-examining these effects. Also, the response to oral therapy may be different from that of the transdermal route, and the methodologies used in the various hemodynamic studies clearly have some impact on the results. As an example, in one study the cerebral blood flow was measured by the sophisticated SPECT technology; an increase in blood flow was demonstrated after only 3 weeks of oral hormone therapy. In contrast, many other investigators failed to show any cardiovascular effect of estrogens within such a limited period of time using echocardiography or plethysmography. Interestingly, preliminary data from our laboratory were somewhat confusing: women who started hormone therapy a few days after surgical castration had a significant decrease in the aortic flow echo parameters 3 weeks later. This was not the case in women undergoing hysterectomy only or in castrated women who did not receive estrogens (unpublished data). Such 'negative' hemodynamic effects were also observed during acute administration of estrogens.

Although intracoronary or intravenous injection of estrogens causes vasodilatation and an increase in arterial and coronary blood flow, we found in the rat heart model that estradiol had a dose-dependent negative chronotropic effect[8]; a negative inotropic effect was recorded when human atrial strips were bathed in estradiol. These effects could be the result of the calcium-blocking property of estrogens, often discussed in the literature[9]. Most studies on acute administration of estrogens in postmenopausal women looked for changes in endothelial function and blood flow[10]. However, there are few studies on LV function and exercise performance in this context. Rosano and colleagues[11] gave sublingual estradiol to postmenopausal women with coronary artery disease. They demonstrated an improvement in exercise testing 40 min post-dose, expressed by prolongation of the time to 1-mm ST depression and the total exercise time, as compared to pre-treatment values. In a similar study, we performed rest and exercise echo-cardiography 1 h after sublingual estradiol had been ingested by the subjects. The resting blood pressure and the peripheral resistance were reduced in 11 postmenopausal women with mild hypertension; also, the aortic blood flow velocity and the size of the left heart cavities decreased. No alterations in flow parameters during exertion were detected[12]. Interestingly, in a study by Leonardo and co-workers[13], using sublingual estradiol at 1 mg and obtaining serum levels of only one-tenth of those of that reported in our study, no changes in resting blood pressure were recorded 20 min post-dose, but the blood flow velocity increased. Sublingual estradiol at 1 mg was also given by Volterrani and colleagues[14], who measured forearm blood flow and peripheral vascular resistance. Despite the estrogen-induced vasodilatation, there were no changes in blood pressure.

In conclusion, although data on the cardiac effects of HRT are mounting rapidly, our knowledge remains incomplete and awaits further clarification.

References

1. Pines A, Fisman EZ, Levo Y, *et al.* Menopause-induced changes in left ventricular wall thickness. *Am J Cardiol* 1992;72:240–41

2. Pines A, Fisman EZ, Drory Y, *et al.* Menopause-induced changes in Doppler-derived parameters of aortic flow in healthy women. *Am J Cardiol* 1992;69:1104–106

3. Eckstein N, Pines A, Fisman EZ, *et al.* The effect of the hypoestrogenic state, induced by gonadotropin-releasing hormone agonist, on Doppler-derived parameters of aortic flow. *J Clin Endocrinol Metab* 1993;77:910–12

4. Celermajer DS, Sorensen KE, Spiegelhalter DJ, *et al.* Aging is associated with endothelial dysfunction in healthy men years before the age-related decline in women. *J Am Coll Cardiol* 1994;24:471–6

5. Malhotra A, Buttrick P, Scheuer J. Effects of sex hormones on development of physiological and pathological cardiac hypertrophy in male and female rats. *Am J Physiol* 1990;259:H866–H871

6. Pines A, Fisman EZ, Ayalon D, *et al.* Long-term effects of hormone replacement therapy on Doppler-derived parameters of aortic flow in postmenopausal women. *Chest* 1992;102:1496–8

7. Pines A, Fisman EZ, Shapira I, *et al.* Exercise echocardiography in postmenopausal hormone users with mild hypertension. *Am J Cardiol* 1996;78:1385–9

8. Eckstein N, Nadler E, Barnea O, *et al.* Acute effects of 17β-estradiol on the rat heart. *Am J Obstet Gynecol* 1994;171:844–8

9. Collins P, Rosano GMC, Jiang C, *et al.* Cardiovascular protection by oestrogen – a calcium antagonist effect? *Lancet* 1993;341:1264–5

10. White MM, Zamudio S, Stevens T, *et al.* Estrogen, progesterone, and vascular reactivity: potential cellular mechanisms. *Endocr Rev* 1995;6:739–51

11. Rosano GMC, Sarrel PM, Poole-Wilson PA, *et al.* Beneficial effect of oestrogen on exercise-induced myocardial ischemia in women with coronary artery disease. *Lancet* 1993;342:133–6

12. Pines A, Fisman EZ, Drory Y, *et al.* The effects of sublingual estradiol on left ventricular function at rest and exercise in postmenopausal women: an echocardiographic study. *Menopause* 1998;5:79–85

13. Leonardo F, Medeirus C, Rosano GMC, *et al.* Effect of acute administration of estradiol 17 beta on aortic blood flow in postmenopausal women. *Am J Cardiol* 1997;80:791–3

14. Volterrani M, Rosano G, Coats A, *et al.* Estrogen acutely increases peripheral blood flow in postmenopausal women. *Am J Med* 1995;99:119–22

Direct vascular effects of ovarian steroids 7

D. de Ziegler

INTRODUCTION

Our belief that ovarian hormones grant women relative protection against cardiovascular diseases stems from the classic epidemiological observation that men have more cardiovascular disease than women of the same age. As early as 1939, Master and colleagues[1] reported that the male sex was a risk factor for myocardial infarction. While other risk factors for coronary heart disease (CHD) are more prone to affect males than females of the same age, attempts at adjusting mortality for the role played by these risk factors have failed to eliminate the sex difference in the prevalence of CHD[2]. The World Health Organization (WHO) data on CHD mortality (Figure 1) showed that the male/female ratio of death from CHD remained remarkably constant over an extremely wide range of CHD prevalence seen in different countries[3]. The WHO report therefore confirmed the observation of McGill and Stern that the magnitude of the sex difference in CHD incidence is a direct function of the prevalence of CHD in the population under study[4].

The primary explanation put forward for the sex difference in the CHD incidence has been the difference in sex hormone patterns. Because the sex difference in CHD incidence vanishes after ovarian function ceases at the time of menopause, it has been envisioned that it is ovarian function that grants women relative protection against CHD. Moreover, because one of the hormones produced by the ovary, estradiol (E_2), has been recognized to induce a favorable alteration of the lipid profile, the entire benefit of ovarian function on CHD incidence has been attributed, possibly too hastily, to the sole effects of E_2[5]. Today we see, however, that both participants in the ovarian function, E_2 and progesterone, are involved in lowering the CHD incidence in women of reproductive age.

Contrasting with the putative beneficial properties of E_2 on the cardiovascular system is the overall consensus obtained from all 19 studies reviewed on plasma E_2 levels and CHD (in men and women) that, contrary to expectations, patients with CHD do not have particularly low estrogen levels. Even more surprising are the findings from 13 of the 19 reviewed studies[6-18] that patients with CHD have elevated E_2 levels, but this was not confirmed by the remaining six authors[19-24]. Several straightforward explanations have been proposed to explain the puzzling observation that high E_2 levels seem to be associated with a higher incidence of CHD. This link appeared to persist after all the attempts made to adjust for each of the possible factors, including body weight[25].

Because ovarian function ceases approximately when the incidence of CHD tends to equal that of men, it has been the objective of hormone replacement therapy (HRT) to extend the relative cardioprotection that women benefit from during their reproductive years. In order to assess the vascular effects of HRT, various parameters have been tested for their ability to reflect the cardioprotective properties of E_2. It is the objective of our present paper to review how certain parameters of the direct effects of ovarian hormones on vessels can serve to monitor the cardioprotective action of HRT and to evaluate the limitation of these possible implications.

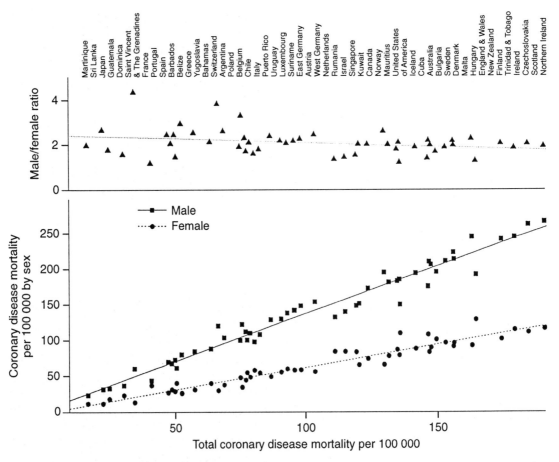

Figure 1 WHO data on coronary heart disease (CHD) mortality in men and women of different countries. Age-standardized coronary disease death rates and ratio of male to female mortality. Despite great differences in CHD death rates between countries, the ratio of male to female mortality is constant at a mean value of 2.24 ± 0.08 (mean ± SEM). Data from World Health Organization, 1987[3]

THE UTERINE ARTERY MODEL

The interest in studying the effects of ovarian hormones on uterine artery blood flow stemmed from the premises that the uterine artery is particularly rich in E_2 receptors (ER) and could therefore represent a privileged territory that provided an amplified reflection of the vascular effects of hormonal preparations. The uterine arteries are identified with color Doppler in the outer layers of the myometrium at the level of the internal os of the cervix. The various branches can be recognized downstream from the entry point of uterine arteries into the uterine muscle. Pulsed Doppler allows determination of an indirect reflection of uterine artery resistance. This is obtained by computing various indices that weigh the respective intensity of maximum and minimum Doppler signals throughout the cardiac cycle. The most commonly used Doppler index in gynecology is the pulsatility index or PI. The higher the PI the higher the impedance to flow in the territory lying downstream from the point of measure. In women deprived of ovarian function either prematurely[26] or at the normal age of menopause[27], pulsed Doppler indicates a high degree of vascular resistance in the uterine artery as expressed by elevated PI values (> 3.5). In both groups of women[26,27], exogenous estrogen treatment induced a prompt decrease in uterine artery PI. The vascular effects of progestins differed, however, from those of progesterone. While synthetic progestins partially cancelled the vasodilatory effects of estrogens[28], progesterone administered transvaginally failed to alter the values of uterine artery PI seen with exposure to E_2 only[26]. A distinct synthetic progestin, nomegestrol acetate, also did not alter the vasodilatory effects of E_2[29]. Further work is needed to determine how these vasodilatory properties of various hormonal preparations compare with the occurrence of CHD.

In a prospective study we investigated 77 women aged 42 to 58 years who consulted while in the pre-, peri- or frankly menopausal state. All women weighed within 10% of their ideal body weight. Women who were still menstruating were studied between cycle days 1 and 10. None had received hormonal treatment for at least 6 weeks prior to their evaluation. The vascular resistance of the uterine arteries was assessed by transvaginal pulsed Doppler using an Acuson 128 machine (Digimed SA, Nyon, Switzerland) equipped with a 5-MHz vaginal probe. Uterine arteries were identified as previously reported on transverse uterine scans conducted at the level of the internal cervical os (Figure 2). Positive recognition of uterine vessels was greatly facilitated by color coding of blood flow. Doppler scans of uterine vessels were verified by repeated measurements of uterine artery Doppler signals obtained after these vessels were identified on the right and left lateral longitudinal scans of the uterus. This latter approach displayed a characteristic division of the ascending uterine artery into anterior and posterior branches. Measurements were conducted on both sides, at the level of the uterine artery trunk and 1 cm downstream from the first ramification of the ascending uterine artery branches. Typical pulsed Doppler recordings obtained in estrogen-deprived women and after 2 weeks of estrogen treatment are illustrated in Figures 3 and 4, respectively. Doppler signals were analyzed

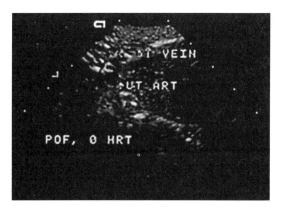

Figure 2 Uterine arteries recognized by Doppler techniques as they enter the uterus at the level of the internal os

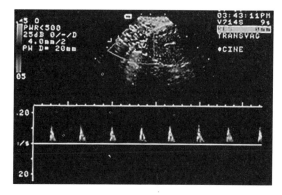

Figure 3 Typical high-impedance pulsed Doppler recording of the uterine artery as observed in a case of estrogen deprivation

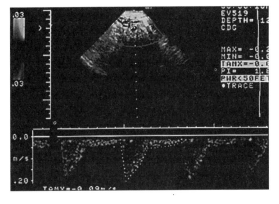

Figure 4 Typical low-impedance pulsed Doppler recording of the uterine artery as observed after 2 weeks only of treatment with exogenous estrogens (Estraderm TTS® 50)

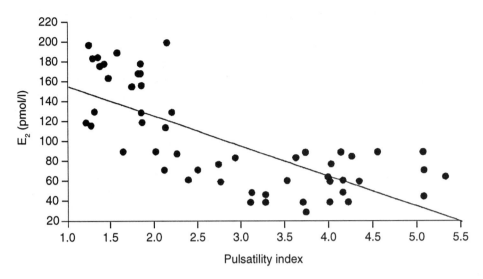

Figure 5 Uterine artery pulsatility index (PI) as a function of plasma estradiol (E_2) levels in women whose plasma E_2 level was ≤ 200 pmol/l (60 pg/ml). In women who had higher E_2 levels, no correlation existed between plasma E_2 levels and uterine artery PI

semiquantitatively by measurement of the PI. Results from each artery were averaged. Blood samples were obtained at the time of Doppler recordings for measurement of plasma levels of E_2 and follicle stimulating hormone (FSH). Correlations between plasma E_2 and PI were studied by linear regression with a range of E_2 values displaying linear correlation with PI on scatter plots.

The precision of Doppler recordings and PI measurements was evaluated by calculating the mean coefficient of variation of multiple measurements ($n = 9$) obtained in seven different women. The precision of repeated PI measurements on the same Doppler recording was 4.2% (inter-Doppler recording variation) while that of repeated Doppler recordings ($n = 9$) obtained on the same vessel in seven other women was 7.8% (inter-Doppler recording variation). Furthermore, comparison of PI measurements obtained in the same person, either on the uterine artery trunk or 1 cm downstream from the first ramification of the ascending uterine branch, did not result in higher inter-Doppler recording variation.

In the present population, the uterine artery PI of frankly menopausal women (E_2

25 pg/ml) was 3.6 ± 0.8, mean $\pm$ SD ($n = 37$), while significantly lower PI measurements (1.5 ± 0.5, mean $\pm$ SD) were obtained in 22 women in whom plasma E_2 exceeded 60 pg/ml ($p < 0.001$). A significant inverse correlation was found between plasma E_2 and PI values ($p < 0.0001$). Scatter plot analysis of plasma E_2 and PI measurements suggested that the inverse correlation was linear when E_2 level was < 60 pg/ml. The linear regression of E_2 over PI is illustrated in Figure 5. While a highly significant inverse correlation existed when E_2 was 60 pg/ml ($p < 0.0001$) none was found between plasma E_2 and uterine artery PI when plasma E_2 was > 60 pg/ml ($n = 22$; $p = 0.7$). Among frankly menopausal women no difference in PI measurement was observed between nulliparous (3.6 ± 1, mean $\pm$ SD), $n = 11$) and multiparous (3.7 ± 0.9, mean $\pm$ SD, $n = 26$) women. Moreover, there was a strong direct correlation between PI and FSH ($p < 0.0001$).

The results of this study of uterine artery PI in perimenopausal women confirmed and extended the results of previous work[26,29] showing that the vascular resistance of uterine arteries is elevated in untreated menopausal women irrespective of whether they are nulliparous or multiparous. In perimenopausal women we observed that the vascular resistance of uterine arteries inversely correlated with plasma E_2 levels when the E_2 level was ≤ 60 pg/ml. In contrast, however, E_2 levels exceeding 60 pg/ml were not associated with a further lowering of uterine artery PI. This is consistent with studies conducted in frankly menopausal women in whom exogenous estrogen given at minimal HRT doses or at the higher 'physiological' amounts used in infertility treatments induced a similar lowering of uterine artery PI. Our original interpretation of these results was that maximum vasodilatation of uterine arteries is achieved by E_2 levels (endogenous or exogenous) lower than mean menstrual cycle levels. While this dose–response pattern resembles that of estrogenic effects on bone resorption, it differs markedly from that of estrogen action on other peripheral markers such as selected liver proteins[30]. In the latter case, liver proteins continue to rise with estrogen exposure increasing above that of the menstrual cycle until maximum stimulation is achieved by E_2 levels in the liver in some cases up to approximately 100 times higher than in the menstrual cycle[30]. We believe today, however, that the vasodilatory response of vessels to estrogen cannot serve for assessing the complete pattern of the dose–response relationship of the E_2 effects on vessels. Indeed, the vasodilatory response to E_2 will itself trigger counter-regulatory phenomena that will limit the expression of the vasodilative properties of E_2 beyond a certain point. Therefore, it cannot be confirmed that the lack of further arterial dilatation with higher E_2 levels equates to no further vascular effects of these higher E_2 levels. This is an inherent limit to the assessment of E_2 effects on vessels by the measurement of the vasodilatory response.

The uterine artery PI may nonetheless prove to be a useful reflector of efficacy for assessing various estrogenic treatments possibly in conjunction with the measurement of endometrial thickness.

Advantages of uterine artery PI measurement over hormonal assays as markers of the efficacy of estrogen treatment include the facts that it provides immediate results, remains unaffected by the pharmacokinetic imperfections of estrogen preparations and remains equally effective for the assessment of estrogenic treatments using not readily measurable estrogens such as ethinyl E_2 or the various components of conjugated equine estrogens (CEE). Verifying the efficacy of estrogen treatments may be clinically indicated in women in whom an accelerated hepatic metabolism of estrogen is feared because of smoking or the use of psychotropic medications (for review, see reference 30) or in women who are at an unusually high risk of osteoporosis or cardiovascular disease.

In infertility, however, uterine artery Doppler data have been reported that appear to contradict this concept that fairly limited levels of E_2 suffice to induce a profound and maximal decrease in uterine artery PI. Indeed, Steer and co-workers[31] showed that nearly half the women undergoing controlled ovarian hyperstimulation (COH) for *in vitro* fertilization (IVF) had an elevated uterine artery PI (> 3.5) on the day of administration of human chorionic gonadotropin (hCG) despite markedly high E_2 levels (≥ 1000 pg/ml) at this stage. Because of similar observations made in women suffering from polycystic ovary disease (high uterine artery PI despite early follicular phase levels of E_2), it has been hypothesized that in certain women the intense ovarian bombardment by human menopausal gonadotropin (hMG) triggers the release by the ovary of a substance that either interferes with the vasodilatory properties of E_2 or exerts vasoactive effects of its own. We refer to this scenario as 'the third factor hypothesis'. Therefore, the apparent paradox between the high E_2 levels of COH and high uterine artery PI seen in some women does not invalidate the clinical value of the uterine artery Doppler approach in menopausal women who are not exposed to these other putative ovarian factors.

NON-INVASIVE ASSESSMENT OF THE ATHEROTIC PROCESS IN THE CAROTID ARTERY

Because of the inherent limitations that hamper the clinical value of assessing the vasodilatory response under different hormonal treatments, interest has focused on new non-invasive approaches for evaluating large vessel wall characteristics as surrogate markers of hormonal effects.

In recent years, B-mode ultrasonography has permitted direct visualization of the superficial arteries and assessment of the vessel wall thickness. In the carotid and femoral artery it is possible to identify two distinct boundaries in the vessel wall: the blood–intima and media–advantice interphases[32]. The distance between these two lines has been defined as the intima–media thickness (IMT). New computer-based systems, such as that proposed by IÔDP, Paris, have been developed that provide an automated measurement of the IMT (Figure 6). It has been proposed that the atherosclerotic process and IMT thickening of the carotid artery parallels plaque deposition in the coronary arteries[32]. In particular, IMT thickening has been associated with an important CHD risk factor, hypercholesterolemia[33–35]. Also, IMT has been associated with age, blood pressure, smoking and diabetes[34,36]. In a study conducted in men, carotid IMT showed a mean increase of 0.12 mm per 2-year interval[37]. While the precision of IMT measurements has been the subject of debate[38] the recent development of automated computer-based approaches has markedly improved the potential usefulness of this method of CHD risk assessment[39]. Figure 6 shows the IMT measured on the common carotid artery with computer-based automated recognition of blood–intima and media–advantice interphases using an expert image analysis system developed by IÔDP medical imaging, Paris. Further work is necessary to determine whether estrogen treatment can limit IMT progression, particularly in women at high risk of CHD, as seen in hypercholesterolemic men receiving

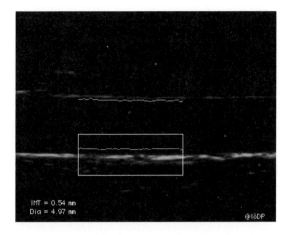

Figure 6 Intima–media thickness measurement in the carotid artery using a computer-based system based on automatic recognition of the blood–intima and media–advantice interphase (IÔDP, Paris)

lipid-lowering therapy[40]. In this study, as illustrated in Figure 7, Mack and colleagues[40] observed a regression of IMT of 0.02 mm/ year in the group receiving active treatment, but this increased by 0.01 mm/year in the individuals who received the placebo[40]. To date, no data exist to confirm or contradict the hypothesis that postmenopausal estrogen treatment can alter the upward trend in IMT measurements observed after women reach menopause. The regression of IMT observed in hypercholesterolemic men receiving specific lipid-lowering treatment is very promising for the clinical value of measuring IMT in menopausal women.

CONCLUSION

Direct measurement of the vasodilatory properties of estrogen treatment has confirmed the importance of the direct effects of hormones. Because of the counter-regulatory mechanisms triggered by the vasodilatory response, this approach does not permit a true study of the dose effect characteristics of the direct effects exerted by estrogens on vessel walls. The recent improvements in the ultrasound-based assessment of IMT and its computer-based

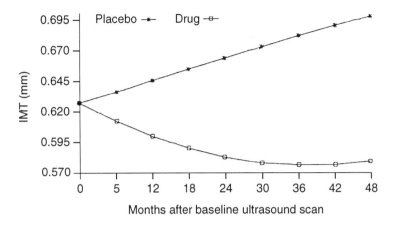

Figure 7 Progression of intima–media thickness (IMT) in hypercholesterolemic men who received placebo or specific lipid-lowering treatment. This observation indicated that a reversibility of IMT with time is very promising for the clinical value of this parameter in the menopause, particularly in individuals at high risk for coronary heart disease

automated measurement in carotid and femoral arteries offers promising prospects for assessing individual responses to estrogen treatments and determining the dose needed to optimize hormonal cardioprotection in women at risk of CHD.

References

1. Master AM, Dack S, Jaffe HL. Age, sex and hypertension in myocardial infarction due to coronary occlusion. *Arch Intern Med* 1939;64:767–86

2. Wingard DL, Suarez L, Barrett-Connor E. The sex differential in mortality from all causes and ischemic heart disease. *Am J Epidemiol* 1983;117:165–72

3. World Health Organization. *1939 – World Health Statistics Annual.* Geneva: WHO, 1987:342–9

4. McGill HC, Stern MP. Sex and atherosclerosis. *Atherosclerosis Rev* 1979;4:157–242

5. Barrett-Connor E, Khaw K-T. Endogenous sex hormones and cardiovascular disease in men. A prospective population-based study. *Circulation* 1988;78:539–45

6. Hauss WH, Junge-Hulsing G, Wagner H, *et al.* Increased 17 beta-estradiol levels in blood of arteriosclerotic patients. *Klin Wochenschr* 1973;51:824–5

7. Wagner H. *Endokrin-metabolische Störungen bei Arteriosklerose.* Stuttgart: Gustave Fisher Verlag, 1975

8. Philips GB. Evidence for hyperoestrogenaemia as a risk factor for myocardial infarction in men. *Lancet* 1976;2:14–18

9. Entrican JH, Beach C, Carroll D, *et al.* Raised plasma oestradiol and oestrone levels in young survivors of myocardial infarction. *Lancet* 1978;2:487–90

10. Levin LC, Korenmann SG. Elevated estradiol levels in acute MI and coronary artery disease. *Clin Res* 1978;26:308A (Abstract).

11. Klaiber EL, Vroverman DM, Haffajee CI, *et al.* Serum estrogen levels in men with acute myocardial infarction. *Am J Med* 1982;73:872–81

12. Labropoulos B, Velonakis E, Oekonomakos P, *et al.* Serum sex hormones in patients with coronary disease and their relationship to known factors causing atherosclerosis. *Cardiology* 1982;69:98–103

13. Luria MH, Johnson MW, Pego R, *et al.* Relationship between sex hormones, myocardial infarction, and occlusive coronary disease. *Arch Intern Med* 1982;142:42–4

14. Winter JH, Wilson GR, Morley KD, *et al.* Estradiol levels in myocardial infarction. *Arch Intern Med* 1982;142:1581–2 [Letter]

15. Small M, Lowe GDO, Beastall GH, *et al.* Serum oestradiol and ischaemic heart disease – relationship with myocardial infarction but not

coronary atheroma or haemostasis. *Q J Med* 1985;57:775–82

16. Aksut SV, Aksut G, Karamehmetoglu A, *et al.* The determination of serum estradiol, testosterone and progesterone in acute myocardial infarction. *Jpn Heart* 1986;27:825–37

17. Srzednicki M, Slowinska-Srzednicka J, Sadowski Z, *et al.* Serum oestradiol level in men with acute myocardial infarction. *Pol Arch Med Wewn* 1986;76:213–21

18. Wilke B, Jaross W, Schollberg K, *et al.* Estradiolspiegel bei Herzinfarktpatienten. *Z Klin Med* 1988;43:621–3

19. Heller RF, Jacobs HS, Vermeulen A, *et al.* Androgens, oestrogens and coronary heart disease. *Br Med J* 1981;282:438–9

20. Zumoff B, Troxler RG, O'Connor J, *et al.* Abnormal hormone levels in men with coronary artery disease. *Arteriosclerosis* 1982;2:58–67

21. Okun M, Fisher ML, Wing L, *et al.* Relationship between serum estradiol and extent of coronary atherosclerosis. *Clin Res* 1985;33:746A (Abstract)

22. Franzen J, Fex G. Low serum apolipoprotein A-I in acute myocardial infarction survivors with normal HDL cholesterol. *Atherosclerosis* 1986;59:37–42

23. Sewdarsen M, Jialal I, Vythilingum S, *et al.* Sex hormone levels in young Indian patients with myocardial infarction. *Arteriosclerosis* 1986;6:418–21

24. Cauley JA, Gutai JP, Kuller LH, *et al.* Usefulness of sex steroid hormone levels in predicting coronary artery disease in men. *Am J Cardiol* 1987;60:771–7

25. Kalin MF, Zumoff B. Sex hormones and coronary disease: a review of the clinical studies. *Steroids* 1990;55:330–52

26. de Ziegler D, Bessis R, Frydman R. Vascular resistance of uterine arteries: physiological effects of estradiol and progesterone. *Fertil Steril* 1991;55:775–9

27. Bourne T, Hillard TC, Whitehead MI, *et al.* Oestrogens, arterial status, and postmenopausal women. *Lancet* 1990;335:1470–1

28. Hillard TC, Bourne TH, Whitehead ME, *et al.* Differential effects of transdermal estradiol and sequential progestogens on impedance to flow within the uterine arteries of postmenopausal women. *Fertil Steril* 1992;58:959–63

29. de Ziegler D, Zartarian M, Micheletti MC, *et al.* L'administration cyclique de Nomégestrol acétate n'altère pas les effets vasodilatateurs de l'estradiol sur l'artère utérine. *Contracept Fertil Sex* 1994;22:767–70

30. de Ziegler D. Is the liver a target organ for estrogen? In Sitruk-Ware R, Utian W, eds. *The Menopause and Replacement Therapy: Facts, Controversies.* New York: Marcel Dekker, 1991:201

31. Steer CV, Campbell S, Tan SL, *et al.* The use of transvaginal color flow imaging after in vitro fertilization to identify optimum uterine conditions before embryo transfer. *Fertil Steril* 1992;57:372–6

32. Baldassarre D, Sci B, Werba JP, *et al.* Common carotid intima–media thickness measurement. *Stroke* 1994;25:1588–92

33. Salonen R, Seppanen K, Rauramaa R, *et al.* Prevalence of carotid atherosclerosis and serum cholesterol levels in eastern Finland. *Arteriosclerosis* 1988;8:788–92

34. Handa N, Matsumoto M, Maeda H, *et al.* Ultrasonic evaluation of early carotid atherosclerosis. *Stroke* 1990;21:1567–72

35. Poli A, Tremoli E, Colomba A, *et al.* Ultrasonagraphic measurement of the common carotid artery wall thickness in hyper-cholesterolemic patients: a new method for the quantitation and follow-up of preclinical atherosclerosis in living human subjects. *Atherosclerosis* 1988;70:253–61

36. Salonen R, Salonen JT. Determinants of carotid intima–media thickness: a population-based ultrasonograph study in eastern Finnish men. *J Intern Med* 1991;229:225–31

37. Salonen R, Salonen JT. Progression of carotid atherosclerosis and its determinants: a population-based ultrasonography study. *Atherosclerosis* 1990;81:33–41

38. Riley WA, Barnes RW, Applegate WB, *et al.* Reproducibility of noninvasive ultrasonic measurement of carotid atherosclerosis: the Asymptomatic Carotid Artery Plaque Study. *Stroke* 1992;23:1062–8

39. Gariepy J, Simon A, Massonneau M, *et al.* Echographic assessment of carotid and femoral arterial structure in men with essential hypertension. *Am J Hypertens* 1996;9:126–36

40. Mack WJ, Selzer RH, Nodis HN, *et al.* One-year reduction and longitudinal analysis of carotid intima–media thickness associated with colestipol/niacin therapy. *Stroke* 1993;24:1779–83

Estrogen deprivation, estrogen replacement and coronary artery atherosclerosis and function: observations on the cynomolgus macaque model

8

T.B. Clarkson

Only since about 1900 have women lived for significant periods beyond the menopause. Currently, women can expect that about one-third of their lifespan will be postmenopausal. The change in life expectancy, relative to the length of time that ovaries produce endogenous estrogen, has led to numerous studies to elucidate the effects of estrogen deprivation on disorders of aging. There is consensus that continued estrogen deprivation results in bone loss with associated fractures, genitourinary dysfunction and progressive coronary artery atherosclerosis, resulting in morbidity and mortality from myocardial ischemia and myocardial infarction. There is also strong evidence (but not yet a consensus) that estrogen deprivation results in declining cognitive function and increased risk for Alzheimer's disease. Because of the limitations of this presentation, comments are restricted primarily to the cardiovascular system, with some comments about brain function.

CHARACTERISTICS OF FEMALE CYNOMOLGUS MONKEYS AS AN ANIMAL MODEL

Cynomolgus monkeys (*Macaca fascicularis*) fed an atherogenic diet develop atherosclerosis with many similarities to the same pathological process of human beings[1,2]. In Figure 1 are listed some lipoprotein and cardiovascular similarities between human beings and female cynomolgus macaques[3].

There are also similarities in reproductive biology. The cynomolgus female has a 28-day menstrual cycle similar to that of women[4]. Furthermore, in cynomolgus females the duration of the follicular and luteal phases, as well as plasma estradiol and progesterone concentrations across the cycle, are remarkably similar to those of women[4,5].

PREMENOPAUSAL ESTROGEN DEFICIENCY AND REPLACEMENT

We have used the cynomolgus macaque model to explore premenopausal situations that might result in a sufficient deficiency of endogenous estrogen to result in patho-physiological changes. The most pronounced finding has been that competitive stress in these monkeys results in ovarian dysfunction, estrogen deficiency, exacerbated coronary artery atherosclerosis and abnormalities in coronary artery vasomotion.

Cynomolgus macaques arrange themselves in a definite social hierarchy: for example, when monkeys are arranged in four-monkey subsets, animals rank one, two, three and four. To be a low-ranked monkey (three or four in the dominance hierarchy of a four-monkey group) is chronically stressful because much time is spent avoiding confrontations with the dominant monkeys. This long-term social stress results in larger adrenal glands, higher plasma cortisol concentrations, ovarian dysfunction (with markedly reduced estradiol production), reduced plasma concentrations

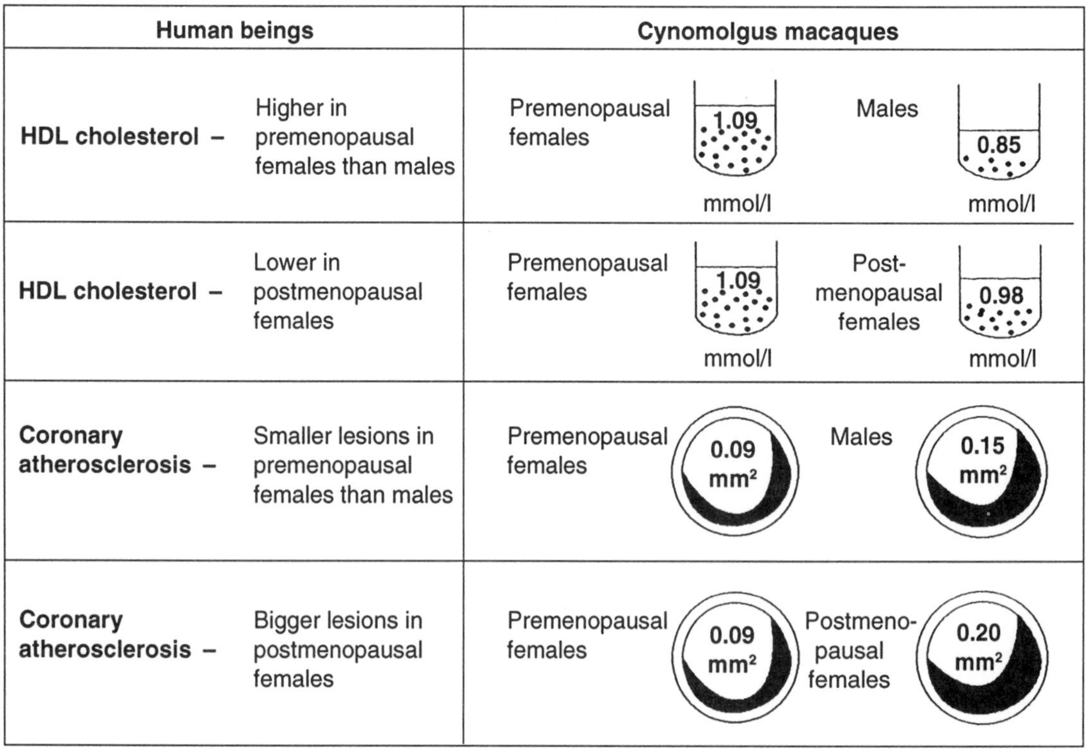

Human beings		Cynomolgus macaques			
HDL cholesterol –	Higher in premenopausal females than males	Premenopausal females	1.09 mmol/l	Males	0.85 mmol/l
HDL cholesterol –	Lower in postmenopausal females	Premenopausal females	1.09 mmol/l	Post-menopausal females	0.98 mmol/l
Coronary atherosclerosis –	Smaller lesions in premenopausal females than males	Premenopausal females	0.09 mm²	Males	0.15 mm²
Coronary atherosclerosis –	Bigger lesions in postmenopausal females	Premenopausal females	0.09 mm²	Postmeno-pausal females	0.20 mm²

Figure 1 Pertinent characteristics of the cynomolgus macaque model compared to humans with respect to high density lipoprotein (HDL) cholesterol concentrations and coronary artery atherosclerosis extent. From Clarkson, 1994[3]

of high density lipoprotein cholesterol (HDL-C), and exacerbated coronary artery atherosclerosis (Figure 2[6]).

These observations suggested to us the potential usefulness of exogenous estrogen treatment for premenopausal females with impaired ovarian function. We tested that hypothesis in a total of 213 premenopausal monkeys fed a moderately atherogenic diet to mimic the typical diet in the USA. They were randomized into two groups, one that received no hormonal treatment and one that received an oral contraceptive (Triphasil®, Wyeth-Ayerst, Princeton, NJ, USA) mixed into the diet[7].

The animals were kept in groups of four or five monkeys, and the social structure within these subgroups was determined weekly. The results showed a reduction of 37% in the extent of iliac artery atherosclerosis in treated animals compared with controls. In accordance with earlier findings, social status significantly predicted atherosclerotic plaque size among control animals; however, among those treated with the oral contraceptive, exacerbated atherosclerosis was prevented in the high-risk low-status categories 3, 4 and 5 (Figure 3).

POSTMENOPAUSAL ESTROGEN DEFICIENCY AND REPLACEMENT

Physiological replacement of ovarian hormones

Many observational studies have found an association between hormone replacement therapy (HRT) and reduced coronary heart disease morbidity and mortality among postmenopausal women (see reference 8 for a meta-analysis). Despite these seemingly convincing findings, it remains controversial

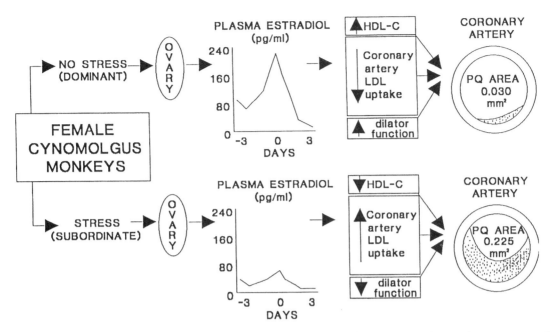

Figure 2 Pathogenetic mechanisms of exacerbated coronary artery atherosclerosis of stressed premenopausal monkeys. From Clarkson *et al.*, 1993[6]

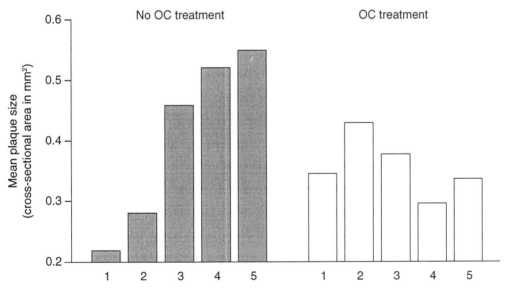

Figure 3 Mean atherosclerosis plaque size in the iliac arteries of premenopausal cynomolgus monkeys with (☐) and without (▨) oral contraceptive (OC) treatment. Numbers under bars represent animals' social status within a five-member group. Adapted from Kaplan *et al.*, 1995[7]

whether cardioprotection reported to occur with postmenopausal replacement of ovarian hormones is a real biological phenomenon or reflects patient selection bias. Researchers have pointed out repeatedly that post-menopausal HRT users are leaner, exercise more, are better educated, have higher incomes and have better access to the medical care system[9-14], any or all of which could reduce the risk of coronary heart disease.

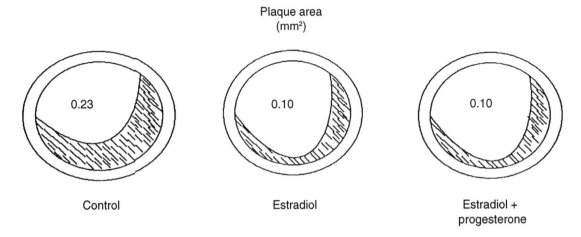

Figure 4 Effect of parental ovarian hormone replacement, 17β-estradiol and 17β-estradiol + progesterone, on coronary artery atherosclerosis in surgically postmenopausal female cynomolgus monkeys. Modified from Adams *et al.*, 1990[15]

To determine the significance, if any, of the patient selection bias, we used surgically postmenopausal cynomolgus monkeys as models for menopausal women in our studies of estrogen replacement effects on coronary artery atherosclerosis. The cynomolgus macaque model has several advantages over retrospective observational studies with women, such as lack of selection bias, adherence to the experimental regimen, better control of potential confounders and availability of pathological endpoints. The monkeys were fed a moderately atherogenic diet to mimic that of the average postmenopausal American woman, and then received either no hormonal treatment, Silastic implants of estradiol (continuous) or estradiol (continuous) plus progesterone (cyclically)[15]. The hormonal treatments had minimal effects on plasma lipid and lipoprotein concentrations. The effect of the treatments on the extent of coronary artery atherosclerosis are shown schematically in Figure 4.

The 50% reduction in the extent of coronary artery atherosclerosis with ovarian hormone replacement is intriguing, since most investigators believe that the reduction in coronary heart disease mortality gained by postmenopausal HRT users is about 50%.

MECHANISMS OF ESTROGEN'S BENEFICIAL EFFECTS ON CORONARY ARTERY ATHEROGENESIS

Plasma lipids and lipoproteins

In further studies of ovarian hormone replacement, we sought to determine what proportion of the beneficial effect on atherogenesis could be ascribed to plasma lipoprotein concentrations, and how much was unknown and presumably associated, at least in part, with changes at the coronary artery wall. Our estimate of the allocation of the beneficial effect on atherogenesis is illustrated schematically in Figure 5.

Coronary artery LDL metabolism

To gain better understanding of some of the plasma lipid-independent mechanisms by which ovarian hormone replacement reduces atherogenesis, we studied arterial uptake of low density lipoprotein (LDL) and coronary artery vasomotion in our monkey model. We measured rates of LDL accumulation within coronary arteries during the early stages of atherogenesis[16]. Use of LDL particles labelled with either of two isotopes enabled us to measure efflux and influx and accumulation

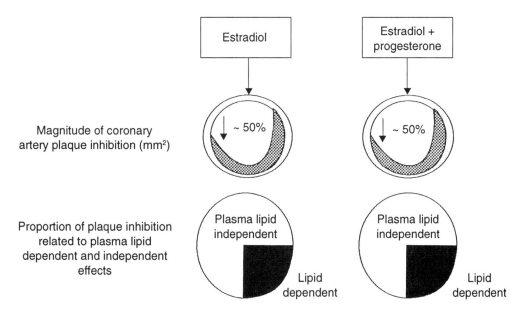

Figure 5 Proportion of plaque-inhibitory effects of ovarian hormone replacement that is plasma lipid dependent and independent. Modified from Adams *et al.*, 1990[15]

of LDL particles within the walls of coronary arteries. The results of one of these studies are illustrated in Figure 6.

Coronary artery LDL uptake in surgically postmenopausal monkeys was increased five- to six-fold over that which occurs in normally cycling premenopausal females[17]. We also noted that the replacement of estradiol plus

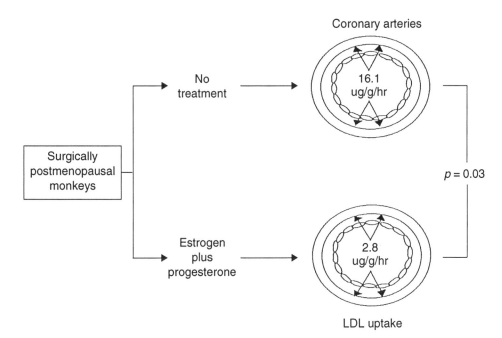

Figure 6 Effects of ovarian hormone replacement (17β-estradiol plus progesterone) on low density lipoprotein (LDL) uptake in the coronary arteries of surgically postmenopausal cynomolgus monkeys. Modified from Wagner *et al.*, 1991[16]

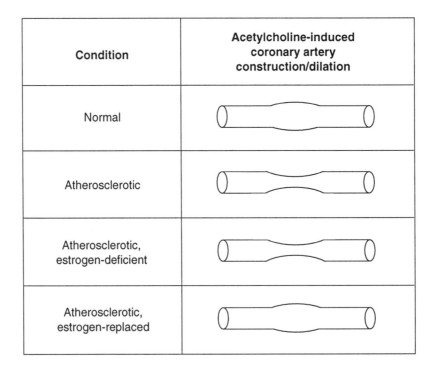

Condition	Acetylcholine-induced coronary artery construction/dilation
Normal	
Atherosclerotic	
Atherosclerotic, estrogen-deficient	
Atherosclerotic, estrogen-replaced	

Figure 7   Effects of atherosclerosis and estrogen replacement therapy on coronary artery vasomotion after acetylcholine infusion in female cynomolgus monkeys. Modified from Williams *et al.*, 1990[18]; 1992[19]

progesterone restored the postmenopausal animals to premenopausal levels of LDL accumulation. We believe that the effect of estradiol on coronary artery LDL metabolism is one of the major mechanisms by which coronary artery atherosclerosis is affected beneficially by estrogen treatment.

Coronary artery vasomotion

Endothelium-dependent vasoconstriction of coronary arteries may promote atherogenesis, especially in association with the adverse effects of nitric oxide depletion on coronary artery cell metabolism. We compared estrogen-deprived atherosclerotic monkeys and estrogen-replaced atherosclerotic monkeys regarding the degree of constriction after intracoronary artery infusion of acetylcholine[18]. Figure 7 is a schematic illustration of the results of those studies.

Treatment of surgically postmenopausal monkeys with estradiol normalized endothelium-dependent vasomotion. This beneficial effect was very prompt, occurring within 20 min after infusion of estradiol[19], and equally prompt after sublingual administration of estrogen in women[20]. The potential atherogenic effects of repeated artery constriction may be considerable and nitric oxide depletion may magnify this effect.

EFFECTS OF MEDROXYPROGESTERONE ACETATE ON CARDIOVASCULAR BENEFITS OF ESTROGEN IN THE MONKEY MODEL

We have examined whether progesterone or a progestin might attenuate some of the protective effect of estrogen against coronary artery atherosclerosis in cynomolgus monkeys. In study 1[15], monkeys were given either no hormone replacement (control), or 17β-estradiol plus cyclic progesterone ($E_2 + P$). These hormones were administered parenterally via Silastic implants to mimic the

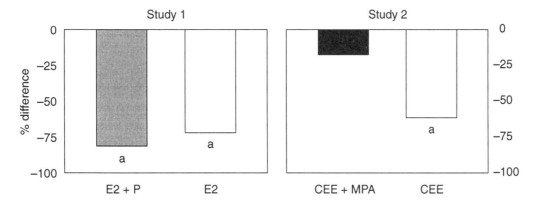

Figure 8 Coronary artery atherosclerosis for two studies of surgically postmenopausal cynomolgus monkeys expressed as the percentage difference in intimal area (plaque size) between the hormone-treated groups and the control group for each study. a, significantly different from control ($p < 0.05$); E2, 17β-estradiol; P, progesterone; CEE, conjugated equine estrogens; MPA, medroxyprogesterone acetate. Study 1 modified from Adams et al., 1990[15]; study 2 modified from Adams et al., 1997[21]

physiological concentrations of circulating estrogen and progesterone. Blank Silastic capsules were implanted in the control group. The estradiol was given continuously and the progesterone was given for 28 days, every other month. In study 2[21], monkeys were given one of the following treatments: no hormone replacement (control); or conjugated equine estrogens (CEE) at a dose equivalent to a woman's dose of 0.625 mg/day; or CEE + continuous medroxyprogesterone acetate (MPA) at a woman's equivalent dose of 2.5 mg/day. The results of both studies are shown in Figure 8. For the hormone-treated groups, coronary artery atherosclerosis is shown as the percentage difference in average intimal area (IA) from the control group for each study.

Natural progesterone and the synthetic progestin MPA differ in their effects on coronary artery atherosclerosis. Although progesterone did not affect the ability of estrogen to inhibit atherosclerosis, MPA significantly diminished its protective effects. Estradiol and CEE had similar effects on the prevention of coronary artery atherosclerosis in these studies. Despite differences between studies in route of administration, type of estrogen and cyclic versus continuous treatment of the progestins, the results are in keeping with the differences in effects on

HDL-C concentrations between these two progestins in the Postmenopausal Estrogen/ Progestin Interventions (PEPI) trial[22], which is discussed in later paragraphs.

FUTURE DIRECTIONS IN HORMONE REPLACEMENT THERAPY

The potential public health impact on morbidity and mortality from coronary heart disease by postmenopausal estrogen therapy has been minimized because the majority of women find the treatment unacceptable. Compliance with postmenopausal HRT has been studied by a number of investigators[9,23–27], and if one averages their estimates of compliance, only about 8% of American women who are naturally menopausal and 55 years or older use HRT.

Ravnikar[14,28] has studied reasons for lack of compliance with HRT among postmenopausal women. Lack of compliance stems primarily from fear of breast cancer and complications related to the necessity of accompanying progestin therapy (i.e. continuing menstrual periods).

To find a regimen of postmenopausal HRT that would be more acceptable to post-menopausal women, we have sought to

Table 1 Target tissue estrogen agonist/antagonist properties of an ideal estrogenic agent

Target tissue	Estrogen action	
	Agonist	Antagonist
Bone	+	−
Brain	+	−
Breast	−	+
Lipoproteins	+	−
Coronary arteries	+	−
Endometrium	−	+
Genitourinary system	+	−

identify alternative postmenopausal treatments with no risk for breast cancer or bone loss, which obviate the need for a progestin and still provide protection against coronary heart disease. We have summarized in Table 1 the characteristics of an ideal estrogenic agent for postmenopausal use. The ideal treatment would provide estrogen agonist effects for the principal cardiovascular risk factors, arteries, bones, brain, and the genitourinary system, while being an estrogen antagonist for the endometrium and mammary glands.

Estrogens and the brain

Our emphasis on potential estrogen-alternative agents being agonist for brain is based on the possibility that postmenopausal estrogen replacement reduces the risk of Alzheimer's disease among aging women, a matter of great national and international interest. Paganini-Hill and Henderson[29] reported the results of a case–control study to assess the influence of postmenopausal HRT on the risk of developing Alzheimer's disease and related dementias. They reported that HRT use was lower among patients with Alzheimer's disease and dementia than among controls (odds ratio 0.69, confidence interval 0.46–1.03). The observation attained conventional statistical significance when the dose of estrogen and length of

postmenopausal estrogen use were considered. The risk of disease decreased both with increasing estrogen dose (test for trend, $p = 0.02$) and increasing duration of use (test for trend, $p = 0.01$).

In another case–control study, Henderson, working with Paganini-Hill and others[30], confirmed that Alzheimer's disease patients were significantly less likely to use estrogen replacement therapy than controls (7% versus 18%). Additionally, Alzheimer's disease patients using estrogen had significantly better scores on a cognitive performance test than non-users (Mini-Mental State Examination scores of 14.9 versus 6.5). Improvements in cognitive function among Alzheimer's patients treated with estrogen have also been confirmed by another group[31-33].

The apparent benefit of estrogen replacement on disorders of brain aging is based on several well-known effects of estrogen on the brain[34-39]. These effects are summarized in Figure 9. The possible relationship between apolipoprotein E accumulation and its role as a matrix for beta-amyloid is speculative at this time, but is based upon several recent and exciting reports[40,41].

We briefly summarize current research on the potential cardiovascular benefits of several alternatives to traditional estrogens.

Raloxifene and droloxifene

Recently, two analogs of tamoxifen have been developed that are of great interest for their potential benefits on the cardiovascular risk of postmenopausal women. The molecular structure of these two compounds, raloxifene and droloxifene, are illustrated in Figure 10. Both compounds have been studied using surgically menopausal rats. A summary of the findings reported in the literature is shown schematically in Figures 11 and 12[42,43].

Both compounds lower total plasma cholesterol (TPC) concentrations, are apparently not uterotrophic and prevent bone loss comparably. In a study of postmenopausal women recently published by Draper and colleagues[44], short-term (8-week) treatment

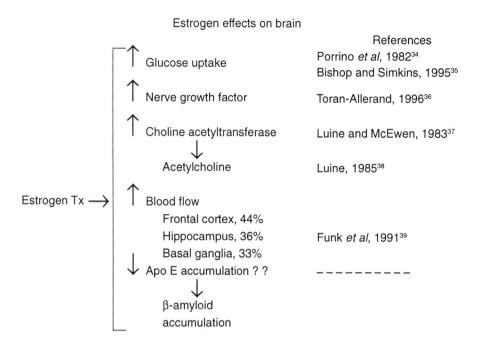

Figure 9 A summary of the known effects of estrogen treatment (Tx) on the brain and their literature citations

with raloxifene (200 mg/day or 600 mg/day) was associated with significant decreases in LDL and TPC concentrations, no change in HDL-C concentrations and increased HDL/LDL ratios. No changes in endometrial tissues were found in either raloxifene group; however, hot flushes were more prevalent in the 600 mg/day group, suggesting a possible estrogen antagonist effect at the level of the brain.

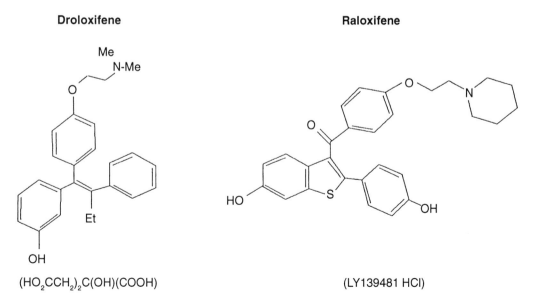

Figure 10 Molecular structures of the compounds droloxifene and raloxifene

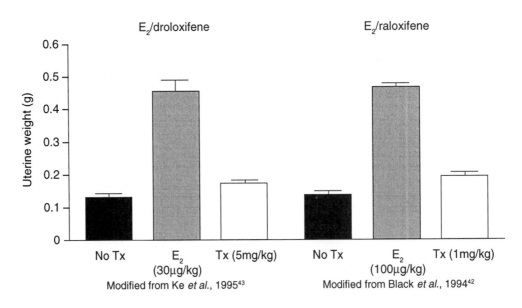

Figure 11 Increases in uterine weight (g) in rats given no treatment (No Tx), estradiol (E_2), or droloxifene (left) or raloxifene (right) treatment

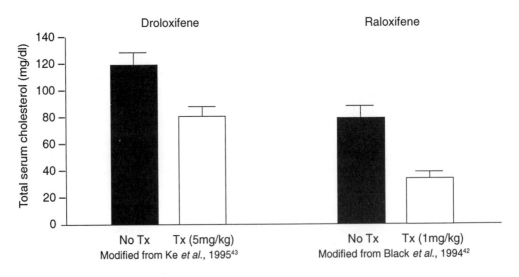

Figure 12 Increases in total serum cholesterol (mg/dl) in rats given no treatment (No Tx), estradiol (E_2), or droloxifene (left) or raloxifene (right) treatment

Whether and to what extent raloxifene shares the antiatherosclerosis properties of estradiol and CEE has been a matter of great interest. Bjarnason and his group[45] have reported on a study of rabbits fed an atherogenic diet and treated with either raloxifene or estradiol. Estradiol had the effect they have reported previously: aorta cholesterols were markedly reduced. Raloxifene treatment had a small effect in reducing aorta cholesterol. More recently, we reported[46] a study comparing the effects on coronary artery atherosclerosis of surgically postmenopausal cynomolgus monkeys fed moderately atherogenic diets and treated with either CEE or raloxifene. CEE treatment resulted in a 70% reduction in coronary artery atherosclerosis, whereas raloxifene had no effect.

Soybean phytoestrogens

We have focused on the phytoestrogens of soybeans as a potential nutritional alternative based upon the putative protective effect of these compounds against the development of breast cancer[47-52] the likely lack of a harmful effect on the uterus[53-59] and an experimental basis for assuming probable favorable effects on coronary artery atherosclerosis, including antioxidant properties[60] and inhibition of smooth muscle cell proliferation[61]. Additionally, a nutritional supplement derived from a natural product may be more acceptable than a pharmacological therapy and thus may improve compliance.

We have compared the effects of CEE and soy bean estrogens on the plasma lipids and lipoproteins of surgically postmenopausal cynomolgus monkeys[62]. In that study, 189 surgically postmenopausal monkeys were randomized into three groups (all fed a moderately atherogenic diet): one group was fed a soy isolate with only trace amounts of genistein and daidzein as the source of dietary protein (Soy(–)); one was fed a soy isolate with the naturally occurring amounts of genistein

and daidzein (1.7 mg/g) (Soy(+)); and one was fed the Soy (–) diet with CEE added at a dose equivalent for a woman of 0.625 mg/day (Soy(–) + CEE). Our preliminary observations are summarized in Table 2. Generally, soy bean phytoestrogen has the same beneficial effects as CEE on the plasma lipids and lipoproteins of postmenopausal monkeys. There are at least two ways in which soy bean phytoestrogen appears to be superior to CEE. First, soy bean phytoestrogen does not result in hypertriglyceridemia, which is consistent with the effect of all mammalian estrogens. Second, soy bean phytoestrogen results in strikingly beneficial increases in concentrations of apolipoprotein A-I.

Both mammalian and synthetic estrogens have been shown to have beneficial effects on coronary artery endothelium-derived relaxation[18,19]. In those experiments, atherosclerotic cynomolgus macaque females were shown to undergo constriction of coronary arteries following acetylcholine infusion. Pretreatment of the animals with estrogen restored their normal endothelium-derived vasomotion, and atherosclerotic female monkeys with pretreatment constriction had normal vasodilation restored. Estrogen is normally combined with a progestin, most commonly MPA in the USA, in postmenopausal hormone replacement. We found that the combined hormone therapy was not as beneficial as estrogen-only

Table 2 A comparison of the effects of soy phytoestrogens (SBE) and of conjugated equine estrogens (CEE) on the plasma lipids and lipoproteins of postmenopausal monkeys (data expressed as percentage of control). Adapted from Anthony et al., 1996[62]

Lipids/lipoproteins	SBE	CEE	p Values SBE vs. CEE
TPC	↓ 16	↓ 17	NS
Triglycerides	↓ 3	↑ 73	< 0.0001
HDL-C	↑ 16	↓ 11	< 0.0001
LDL+VLDL-C	↓ 22	↓ 19	NS
TPC:HDL-C	↓ 30	↑ 2	0.005
Lp(a)	↓ 8	↓ 11	NS
Apo A-1	↑ 14	↓ 5	0.0001

HDL-C, high density lipoprotein cholesterol; LDL, low density lipoprotein; TPC, total plasma cholesterol; VLDL-C, very low density lipoprotein cholesterol

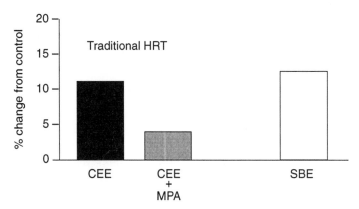

Figure 13 Effects of conjugated equine estrogens (CEE), combined hormone replacement therapy (HRT) in the form of CEE plus medroxyprogesterone acetate (CEE + MPA), and dietary soybean estrogens (SBE) on coronary artery reactivity, expressed as percentage change in dilation versus control, in surgically postmenopausal cynomolgus monkeys. Adapted from Williams *et al.*, 1994[63] and Honoré *et al.*, 1998[64]

therapy on the vasodilatation of athero-sclerotic coronary arteries[63]. Thus, the progestin in the usual hormone replacement antagonized the benefits of estrogen. We have viewed the therapeutic effect of estrogen as an indicator of estrogen agonist effects on the coronary arteries, and thus have sought to determine how soy bean phytoestrogens compared with estrogen-only and combined hormone replacement on coronary artery vasomotion.

In Figure 13 we summarize the results of two experiments in which atherosclerotic female monkeys were treated with CEE (estrogen-only), CEE + MPA (combined hormone replacement), or soy bean phytoestrogens (Soy (+))[64]. These data suggest to us an estrogen agonist effect of soy bean phytoestrogens on coronary arteries that is comparable to that of CEE, and that both these treatments are superior to the usual combined hormone replacement regimen of CEE plus MPA.

OTHER POTENTIAL SELECTIVE ESTROGEN RECEPTOR MODULATORS

A 1.5% component of CEE, 17α-dihydroequilenin (DHEN), has been shown by our group to have interesting target tissue-specific estrogen agonist effects. We observed that DHEN markedly reduced plasma cholesterol concentrations in ovariectomized rats without causing uterine hyperplasia[65]. In both male and female rhesus monkeys, DHEN prevented paradoxical coronary artery vasoconstriction to infusion of acetylcholine[66]. In the males, treatment with DHEN was associated with a 60% reduction in arterial accumulation of LDL. We saw no evidence of reproductive tract abnormalities in either males or females. More recently, Washburn and coworkers[67] presented evidence that DHEN was equivalent to estradiol in maintaining dendritic spine densities of brains of estrogen-deprived rats while having no uterotrophic effect.

SUMMARY

Estrogen replacement therapy for post-menopausal women is associated with marked decreases in morbidity and mortality from coronary heart disease. The therapeutic benefits of estrogens on coronary heart disease have been shown to be minimally related to their beneficial effects on plasma lipids and lipoproteins; instead, they derive primarily from the direct effects of estrogens on the coronary arteries.

The potential public health impact of estrogen replacement therapy has not been realized because of poor compliance (about 8% of naturally menopausal American women beyond age 55). Poor compliance stems in large part from fear of breast cancer and the disadvantages associated with the necessity of combining a progestin to prevent endometrial cancer. Research concerning estrogen replacement therapy is being directed toward therapies that may be first, as beneficial as traditional estrogens for bone, brain and the cardiovascular system; second, estrogen antagonists for breast and endometrium; and third, well tolerated without a progestin.

ACKNOWLEDGEMENT

This work was supported in part by Grant P01HL45666, National Heart, Lung and Blood Institute, National Institutes of Health, Bethesda, MD, USA.

References

1. Kramsch DM, Hollander W. Occlusive atherosclerotic disease of the coronary arteries in monkeys (*Macaca irus*) induced by diet. *Exp Mol Pathol* 1968;9:1–9

2. Stary HC, Malinow MR. Ultrastructure of experimental coronary artery atherosclerosis. *Atherosclerosis* 1982;43:151–75

3. Clarkson TB. Estrogens, progestins and coronary heart disease in cynomolgus monkeys. *Fertil Steril* 1994;62(Suppl 2):147S–151S

4. Williams RF, Hodgen GD. The reproductive cycle in female macaques. *Am J Primatol* 1982;1(Suppl 1):181–92

5. Adams MR, Kaplan JR, Clarkson TB, et al. Ovariectomy, social status, and atherosclerosis in cynomolgus monkeys. *Arteriosclerosis* 1985;5:192–200

6. Clarkson TB, Adams MR, Williams JK, et al. Clinical implications of animal models of gender difference in heart disease. In Douglas PS, ed. *Cardiovascular Health and Disease in Women.* Philadelphia: WB Saunders, 1993:283–302

7. Kaplan JR, Adams MR, Anthony MS, et al. Dominant social status and contraceptive hormone treatment inhibit atherogenesis in premenopausal monkeys. *Arterioscler Thromb Vasc Biol* 1995;15:2094–100

8. Stampfer MJ, Colditz GA. Estrogen replacement therapy and coronary heart disease: a quantitative assessment of the epidemiologic evidence. *Prevent Med* 1991;20:47–63

9. Derby CA, Hume AL, Barbour MM, et al. Correlates of postmenopausal estrogen use and trends through the 1980s in two southeastern New England communities. *Am J Epidemiol* 1993;137:1125–35

10. Stampfer MJ, Colditz GA, Willett WC, et al. Postmenopausal estrogen therapy and cardiovascular disease. Ten-year follow-up from the Nurses' Health Study. *N Engl J Med* 1991;325:756–62

11. Criqui MH, Suarez L, Barrett-Connor E, et al. Postmenopausal estrogen use and mortality. Results from a prospective study in a defined, homogeneous community. *Am J Epidemiol* 1988;128:606–14

12. Barrett-Connor E, Wingard DL, Criqui MH. Postmenopausal estrogen use and heart disease risk factors in the 1980s: Rancho Bernardo, Calif, revisited. *J Am Med Assoc* 1989;261:2095–2100

13. Rosenberg L, Shapiro S, Kaufman DW, et al. Patterns and determinants of conjugated estrogen use. *Am J Epidemiol* 1979;109:676–86

14. Ravnikar VA. Compliance with hormone therapy. *Am J Obstet Gynecol* 1987;156:1332–4

15. Adams MR, Kaplan JR, Manuck SB, et al. Inhibition of coronary artery atherosclerosis by 17-beta estradiol in ovariectomized monkeys: lack of an effect of added progesterone. *Arteriosclerosis* 1990;10:1051–7

16. Wagner JD, Clarkson TB, St Clair RW, et al. Estrogen and progesterone replacement therapy reduces low density lipoprotein accumulation in the coronary arteries of surgically post-menopausal cynomolgus monkeys. *J Clin Invest* 1991;88:1995–2002

17. Wagner JD, Adams MR, Schwenke DC, et al. Oral contraceptive treatment decreases arterial low density lipoprotein degradation in female cynomolgus monkeys. *Circ Res* 1993;72:1300–307

18. Williams JK, Adams MR, Klopfenstein HS. Estrogen modulates responses of atherosclerotic coronary arteries. *Circulation* 1990;81:1680–7

19. Williams JK, Adams MR, Herrington DM, et al. Effects of short-term estrogen treatment on vascular responses of coronary arteries. *J Am Coll Cardiol* 1992;20:452–7

20. Rosano GMC, Sarrel PM, Poole-Wilson PA, *et al.* Oestrogen improves exercise-induced myocardial ischaemia in female patients with coronary artery disease. *Lancet* 1993;342:133–6

21. Adams MR, Register TC, Golden DL, *et al.* Medroxyprogesterone acetate antagonizes inhibitory effects of conjugated equine estrogens on coronary artery atherosclerosis. *Arterioscler Thromb Vasc Biol* 1997;17:217–21

22. Writing Group for the PEPI Trial. Effects of estrogen or estrogen/progestin regimens on heart disease risk factors in postmenopausal women. The Postmenopausal Estrogen/ Progestin Interventions (PEPI) Trial. *J Am Med Assoc* 1995;273:199–208

23. Bush TL, Cowan LD, Barrett-Connor E, *et al.* Estrogen use and all-cause mortality. Preliminary results from the Lipid Research Clinics Program Follow-Up Study. *J Am Med Assoc* 1983;249:903–6

24. Standeven M, Criqui MH, Klauber MR, *et al.* Correlates of change in postmenopausal estrogen use in a population-based study. *Am J Epidemiol* 1986;124:268–74

25. Egeland GM, Matthews KA, Kuller LH, *et al.* Characteristics of noncontraceptive hormone users. *Prevent Med* 1988;17:403–11

26. Hemminski E, Brambilla DJ, McKinlay SM, *et al.* Use of estrogens among middle-aged Massa-chusetts women. *Ann Pharmacother* 1991;25:418–22

27. Nabulsi AA, Folsom AR, White A, *et al.*, for the ARIC Investigators. Association of hormone-replacement therapy with various cardiovascular risk factors in postmenopausal women. *N Engl J Med* 1993;328:1069–75

28. Ravnikar VA. Compliance with hormone replacement therapy: are women receiving the full impact of hormone replacement therapy's preventive health benefits? *Women's Health Issues* 1992;2:75–82

29. Paganini-Hill A, Henderson VW. Estrogen deficiency and risk of Alzheimer's disease in women. *Am J Epidemiol* 1994;140:256–61

30. Henderson VW, Paganini-Hill A, Emanuel CK, *et al.* Estrogen replace-ment therapy in older women. Comparisons between Alzheimer's disease cases and nonde-mented control subjects. *Arch Neurol* 1994;51:896–900

31. Ohkura T, Isse K, Akazawa K, *et al.* Evaluation of estrogen treatment in female patients with dementia of the Alzheimer's type. *Endocrine J* 1994;41:361–71

32. Ohkura T, Isse K, Akazawa K, *et al.* Long-term estrogen replacement therapy in female patients with dementia of the Alzheimer type: 7 case reports. *Dementia* 1995;6:99–107

33. Ohkura T, Isse K, Akazawa K, *et al.* Low-dose estrogen replacement therapy for Alzheimer disease in women. *Menopause* 1994;1:125–30

34. Porrino LJ, Nehlig A, Namba H, *et al.* Modulation of local cerebral glucose metabolism by estrogen and progesterone in the hypo-thalamus of ovariectomized female rats. *Soc Neurosci Abstract* 8:1982

35. Bishop J, Simpkins JW. Estradiol enhances brain glucose uptake in ovariectomized rats. *Brain Res Bull* 1995;36:315–20

36. Toran-Allerand CD. The estrogen/neurotrophin connection during neural development: is co-localization of estrogen receptors with the neutrophins and their receptors biologically relevant. *Dev Neurosci* 1996;18:36–48

37. Luine VN, McEwen BJ. Sex differences in cholinergic enzymes of diagonal band nuclei inthe rat preoptic area. *Neuroendocrinology* 1983;36:475–82

38. Luine VN. Estradiol increases choline acetyltransferase activity in specific basal forebrain nuclei and projection areas in female rats. *Exp Neurol* 1985;89:484–90

39. Funk JL, Mortel KF, Meyer JS. Effects of estrogen replacement therapy in cerebral perfusion and cognition among postmenopausal women. *Dementia* 1991;2:268–72

40. Sparks DL, Scheff SW, Hunsaker JC III, *et al.* Induction of Alzheimer-like β-amyloid immunoreactivity in the brains of rabbits with dietary cholesterol. *Exp Neurol* 1994;126:88–94

41. Sparks DL, Liu H, Gross DR, *et al.* Increased density of cortical apolipoprotein E immuno-reactive neurons in rabbit brain after dietary administration of cholesterol. *Neurosci Lett* 1995;187:142–44

42. Black LJ, Sato M, Rowley ER, *et al.* Raloxifene (LY139481) HCl prevents bone loss and reduces serum cholesterol without causing uterine hypertrophy in ovariectomized rats. *J Clin Invest* 1994;93:63–9

43. Ke HZ, Simmons HA, Pirie CM, *et al.* Droloxifene, a new estrogen antagonist/agonist, prevents bone loss in ovariectomized rats. *Endocrinology* 1995;136:2435–41

44. Draper MW, Flowers DE, Huster WJ, *et al.* A controlled trial of raloxifene (LY139481) HCl: impact on bone turnover and serum lipid profile in healthy postmenopausal women. *J Bone Miner Res* 1996;11:835–42

45. Bjarnason NH, Haarbo J, Byrjalsen I, *et al.* Raloxifene inhibits aortic accumulation of cholesterol in ovariectomized, cholesterol-fed rabbits. *Circulation* 1997;96:1964–9

46. Clarkson TB, Anthony MS, Jerome CP. Lack of effect of raloxifene on coronary artery atherosclerosis of postmenopausal monkeys. *J Clin Endocrinol Metab* 1998;83:721–6

47. Adlercreutz H. Western diet and Western diseases: some hormonal and biochemical mechanisms and associations. *Scand J Lab Clin Invest* 1990;50(Suppl 201):3–23

48. Coward L, Barnes NC, Setchell KDR, *et al.* Genistein, daidzein, and their β-glycoside conjugates: antitumor isoflavones in soybean

foods from American and Asian diets. *J Agr Food Chem* 1993;41:1961–7

49. Adlercreutz H, Hämäläinen E, Gorbach S, *et al*. Dietary phyto-oestrogens and the menopause in Japan [letter]. *Lancet* 1992;339:1233

50. Barnes S, Peterson G, Grubbs C, *et al*. Potential role of dietary isoflavones in the prevention of cancer. In Jacobs MM, ed. *Diet and Cancer: Markers, Prevention, and Treatment*. New York: Plenum Press, 1994:135–47

51. Clarkson TB, Anthony MS, Hughes CL Jr. Estrogenic soybean isoflavones and chronic disease: risks and benefits. *Trends Endocrinol Metab* 1995;6:11–16

52. Knight DC, Eden JA. Phytoestrogens – a short review. *Maturitas* 1995;22:167–75

53. Bennets HW, Underwood EJ, Shier FL. A specific breeding problem of sheep on subterranean clover pasture in Western Australia. *Austr Vet J* 1946;22:2–12

54. Bradbury RB, White DE. The chemistry of subterranean clover. Part I. Isolation of formononetin and genistein. *J Chem Soc* 1951;30:3447–9

55. Cheng E, Story CD, Yoder L, *et al*. Estrogenic activity of isoflavone derivatives extracted and prepared from soybean oil meal. *Science* 1953;118:164–5

56. Setchell KDR, Gosselin SJ, Welsh MB, *et al*. Dietary estrogens – a probable cause of infertility and liver disease in captive cheetahs. *Gastroenterology* 1987;93:225–33

57. Bickoff EM, Livingston AL, Hendrickson AP, *et al*. Relative potencies of several estrogen-like compounds found in forages. *J Agr Food Chem* 1993;41:1961–7

58. Baird DD, Umbach DM, Lansdell L, *et al*. Dietary intervention study to assess estrogenicity of dietary soy among postmenopausal women. *J Clin Endocrinol Metab* 1995;80:1685–1690

59. Cline JM, Soderqvist G, von Schoultz E, *et al*. Effects of hormone replacement therapy on the mammary gland of surgically postmenopausal cynomolgus macaques. *Am J Obstet Gynecol* 1996;174:93–100

60. Wei H, Wei L, Frenkel K, *et al*. Inhibition of tumor promoter induced hydrogen peroxide formation *in vitro* and *in vivo* by genistein. *Nutr Cancer* 1993;20:1–12

61. Fujio Y, Yamada F, Takahashi K, *et al*. Responses of smooth muscle cells to platelet-derived growth factor are inhibited by herbimycin – a tyrosine kinase inhibitor. *Biochem Biophys Res Commun* 1993;195:79–83

62. Anthony MS, Clarkson TB, Hughes CL Jr, *et al*. Soybean isoflavones improve cardiovascular risk factors without affecting the reproductive system of peripubertal rhesus monkeys. *J Nutr* 1996;126:43–50

63. Williams JK, Honoré EK, Washburn SA, *et al*. Effects of hormone replacement therapy on reactivity of atherosclerotic coronary arteries in cynomolgus monkeys. *J Am Coll Cardiol* 1994;24:1757–61

64. Honoré EK, Williams JK, Clarkson TB. Soy isoflavones enhance coronary vascular reactivity in atherosclerotic female macaques. *Fertil Steril* 1997;67:148–54

65. Washburn SA, Adams MR, Clarkson TB, *et al*. A conjugated equine estrogen with differential effects on uterine weight and plasma cholesterol in the rat. *Am J Obstet Gynecol* 1993;169:251–6

66. Washburn SA, Honoré EK, Cline JM, *et al*. Effects of 17α-dihydroequilenin sulfate on atherosclerotic male and female rhesus monkeys. *Am J Obstet Gynecol* 1996;175:341–51

67. Washburn SA, Lewis CE, Johnson JE, *et al*. 17α-Dihydroequilenin increases hippocampal dendritic spine density of ovariectomized rats. *Brain Res* 1997;758:241–4

Anti-ischemic effect of 17β-estradiol in menopausal women with coronary artery disease

9

G.M.C. Rosano, F. Leonardo and S.L. Chierchia

INTRODUCTION

The incidence of ischemic cardiovascular events in women before the age of natural menopause is negligible[1]. After the natural menopause, however, this incidence increases and in a few years it becomes similar to that of the male population of similar age[2]. The results of epidemiological studies have shown that young women undergoing bilateral oophorectomy have an incidence of cardiovascular disease similar to that of men of similar age and that menopausal women receiving estrogen replacement therapy have an approximately 50% reduction of coronary events compared to non-users. These observations have led to the suggestion that estrogen deficiency may play a role in the development of coronary artery disease in women and that estrogen replacement therapy has protective effects upon the cardiovascular system[3]. Several different mechanisms have been described to explain these effects[4]. The fact that estrogens decrease total serum cholesterol and, more importantly, low-density lipoprotein (LDL) cholesterol, has led to the suggestion that most of the reduction in cardiovascular mortality and morbidity produced by these hormones is dependent upon this effect[5]. However, more recent evidence suggests that other mechanisms may play an equally important role. Indeed, estrogens directly inhibit the development of atherosclerosis and play a pivotal role in the maintenance of arterial hemodynamics. Estrogens in general and 17β-estradiol in particular are vasoactive substances. They increase cardiac output and arterial blood flow velocity and decrease systemic vascular resistances[6]. *In vitro*, 17β-estradiol causes marked vasodilatation, possibly via a calcium antagonistic mechanism; i*n vivo* it reverses the acetylcholine-induced vasoconstriction observed in animal and human atheromatous vessels[7], possibly through an endothelium-mediated mechanism.

Therefore, the increased incidence of coronary artery disease observed after the menopause, apart from being the consequence of the progression of coronary atherosclerosis, may also be caused by the reduction of the coronary and peripheral vasodilator reserve that results from decreased production of ovarian hormones. Since 17β-estradiol has been shown to dilate both peripheral and coronary arteries in humans[8,9], estrogens should affect coronary flow reserve and myocardial oxygen consumption and therefore may beneficially affect myocardial ischemia.

EFFECT OF ESTROGENS ON EXERCISE-INDUCED MYOCARDIAL ISCHEMIA

Rosano and co-workers[10] have shown that the acute administration of 17β-estradiol delays the onset of exercise-induced myocardial ischemia in menopausal women with coronary artery disease. These authors studied 11 patients with angiographically proven coronary artery disease and exercise-induced myocardial ischemia. After a run-in exercise

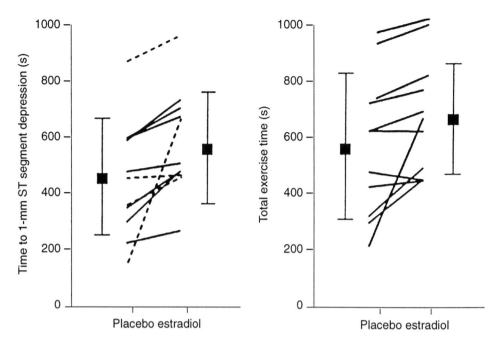

Figure 1 Effect of 17β-estradiol on time to 1-mm ST segment depression and total exercise time in female patients with coronary artery disease. Broken lines indicate patients who, after estradiol administration, did not achieve 1-mm ST segment depression. Reproduced with permission from Rosano *et al.*, 1993[10]

evaluation, patients underwent two exercise tests on 2 different days, 40 min after the sublingual administration of either 17β-estradiol (1 mg) or placebo, given in random order. All patients experienced chest pain and had at least 1 mm ST segment depression on the electrocardiogram (ECG) during the exercise test performed after placebo. However, only seven had ischemia and six experienced chest pain during the test performed after sublingual 17β-estradiol. Furthermore, compared to placebo, 17β-estradiol increased the level of heart rate recorded at the onset of ischemia, the time to 1-mm ST segment depression and total exercise duration (Figure 1). Patients with lower baseline plasma levels of 17β-estradiol showed a greater improvement in exercise-induced ischemia, whereas two patients with the highest plasma concentrations of the hormone had the smallest increase in time to 1-mm ST segment depression. The anti-ischemic effect induced by 17β-estradiol was similar to that observed after acute administration of sublingual nitrates. Although well within the physiological (mid-cycle) range, the plasma levels of 17β-estradiol achieved in the latter study during the active drug phase (2531 pmol/l) were significantly higher that those achieved during chronic replacement therapy. This raises the question of whether 17β-estradiol plasma levels achieved during chronic replacement therapy exert similar anti-ischemic effects. The results obtained by Rosano have been questioned by two recent investigations. Holdright and colleagues[11] found no effect of 48-h admini-stration of 17β-estradiol (patches) on exercise test parameters in female menopausal patients with coronary artery disease. The plasma levels of 17β-estradiol achieved during the acute estrogen phase were in the upper level of the menopausal range and therefore inadequate to have any effect upon cardio-vascular hemodynamics. More recently, Al-Khalili and colleagues[12] were unable to show any anti-ischemic effect after giving 2 mg of 17β-estradiol sublingually to 12 postmenopausal women with coronary artery disease. In this study, however, the plasma levels of 17β-estradiol achieved after dosing were supraphysiological (> 6000 pmol/l), and, of noteworthy importance, not all patients were in pharmacological wash-out and more than a half of them were on active anti-ischemic therapy with β-blockers. Interestingly, a significant improvement in exercise-induced myocardial ischemia was noted after acute administration of sublingual nitrates compared to placebo, but no significant difference between nitrates and 17β-estradiol was detected. Furthermore, the degree of ST segment depression during exercise and the total exercise time were not affected by either nitrates and or 17β-estradiol, suggesting that β-blockade greatly influenced the exercise test response.

EFFECT OF ESTROGENS ON PACING-INDUCED MYOCARDIAL ISCHEMIA

Evaluation of myocardial ischemia by the exercise ECG carries some relevant limitations that prevent the assessment of the severity and the exact timing of its onset. The demonstration of a shift towards a more acidic pH in the blood of the coronary sinus is correlated with the shift from aerobic to anaerobic metabolism in the myocyte and represents an accurate marker of myocardial ischemia[13–15]. Recently, by monitoring the coronary sinus pH in female menopausal patients with coronary artery disease, we showed[16] that sublingual administration of 17β-estradiol (1 mg) improved pacing-induced myocardial schemia. We studied 16 menopausal women referred for cardiac catheterization because of symptoms suggesting ischemic heart disease with significant stenosis of the left anterior descending coronary artery. They underwent continuous monitoring of the coronary sinus pH in control conditions and during incremental atrial pacing (up to 160 bpm). They were then randomized to receive either 17β-estradiol (1 mg sublingually; nine patients) or sublingual placebo (seven patients) 20 min before a second pacing was

performed. Compared to placebo, 17β-estradiol significantly increased the time to onset of myocardial ischemia during pacing and the degree of pH shift at peak pacing. The plasma levels of 17β-estradiol rose to 426 ± 89 pmol/l in patients receiving 17β-estradiol. The results of this study confirmed our early observations[10] showing that the sublingual administration of 17β-estradiol improves exercise-induced myocardial ischemia in a similar patient population. In the latter study, however, the plasma levels of 17β-estradiol were significantly lower than those observed in the exercise study and similar to those usually achieved during estrogen replacement therapy.

POSSIBLE MECHANISMS

The anti-ischemic effects observed after acute administration of 17β-estradiol probably result from both coronary and peripheral vasodilatation which is partially mediated by the vascular endothelium but also by a direct effect of the hormone upon the smooth muscle cells. Jiang and co-workers[7] suggested that 17β-estradiol relaxes coronary arteries *in vitro* by an endothelium-independent mechanism which may be related to the calcium antagonistic properties of the hormone. Collins and associates[17] showed that intracoronary administration of 17β-estradiol in women with coronary artery disease reverts the vasoconstrictor response to acetylcholine to vasodilatation and suggested that the effect is mediated by endothelial cell nitric oxide production. Their conclusion is also supported by the recent finding[18] of enhanced nitric oxide production by human endothelial cells exposed to 17β-estradiol for 20–30 min. We have recently reported that intracoronary infusion of 17β-estradiol attenuates the vasoconstrictor response to methylergometrine in menopausal patients with coronary artery disease[19]. This effect, which may be due to the calcium antagonistic properties of the hormone, may be relevant in those patients in whom an augmented coronary vasomotor tone plays an important role in the development of myocardial ischemia. 17β-estradiol may also prevent myocardial ischemia by reducing myocardial oxygen consumption through a decrease in peripheral vascular resistance or by lowering the preload. Animal studies have shown that the administration of 17β-estradiol leads to increased cardiac output, increased aortic flow velocity, decreased vascular resistance and decreased systolic and diastolic blood pressure[6]. Human studies have reported an estrogen-induced increase in blood flow in the vagina, vulva and uterine and carotid vessels[8]. Acute administration of 17β-estradiol also reduces peripheral vascular resistance in menopausal women[9]. Animal and human studies[17,20-23] suggest that 17β-estradiol may induce vasodilatation by stimulating endothelium-dependent relaxation, possibly by promoting the release of endothelium-derived relaxing factor (EDRF). While that mechanism remains possible, there appears to be a variety of ways in which the hormone can influence vasomotor control. For example, estrogens have an effect upon the sympathetic tone, as these hormones influence the release and uptake of epinephrine (adrenaline) and norepinephrine (noradrenaline) at pre-synaptic junctions[24,25]. Estrogens have also been shown to affect the release of histamine, 5-hydroxytryptamine, dopamine and vasoactive intestinal peptide, all substances which have vasoactive properties and which may influence coronary flow reserve[25-27]. In hypoestrogenic states, disruption of the autonomic control of the cardiovascular system leads to vasomotor instability, as evidenced by sudden increases in serum epinephrine and norepinephrine concentrations when women have hot flushes[28,29]. Estrogen replacement therapy is extremely effective in restoring vasomotor stability and possibly does so by controlling the release of catecholamines[25,30,31]. Indeed, we have recently shown[31] that estrogen replacement therapy normalizes the altered neural control of the cardiovascular system in menopausal women. As increased sympathetic tone may reduce coronary flow reserve, the normalization of the cardiovascular autonomic control may also contribute to the anti-ischemic effect of these hormones. However, the plasma levels of 17β-estradiol achieved during optimal hormone replacement therapy may be slightly lower than those achieved by the acute administration employed by most studies; therefore, it is possible that the anti-ischemic effect seen in these studies may not be as prominent during chronic therapy. On the other hand, long-term administration of 17β-estradiol may also result in other unidentified beneficial cardiovascular effects that may improve outcome and quality of life.

In conclusion, acute systemic administration of 17β-estradiol improves myocardial ischemia in female menopausal patients with coronary artery disease. This effect seems to be dependent upon both coronary and peripheral vascular effects. Studies are needed in order to establish whether the effects seen in acute therapy are sustained during chronic therapy.

References

1. Colditz GA, Willett WC, Stampfer MJ, *et al.* Menopause and the risk of coronary heart disease in women. *N Engl J Med* 1987;316:1105–10
2. Kannel WB, Hjortland MC, McNamara PM, *et al.* Menopause and the risk of cardiovascular disease: the Framingham study. *Ann Int Med* 1976;85:447–52
3. Bush TL, Barrett-Connor E, Cowan LD, *et al.* Cardiovascular mortality and noncontraceptive use of estrogen in women: results from the Lipid Research Clinics Program Follow-up Study. *Circulation* 1987;75:1102–109
4. Gerhard M, Ganz P. How do we explain the clinical benefit of estrogen? From bedside to bench. *Circulation* 1995;92:5–8
5. Bush TL. Noncontraceptive estrogen use and cardiovascular disease. *Epidemiol Rev* 1985;7:80–104

6. Magness RR, Rosenfeld CR. Local and systemic estradiol 17 beta: effects on uterine and systemic vasodilation. *Am J Physiol* 1989;256:E536- E542

7. Jiang C, Sarrel PM, Lindsay DC, *et al.* Endothelium-independent relaxation of rabbit coronary artery by 17β-estradiol *in vitro. Br J Pharmacol* 1991;104:1033–7

8. Killam AP, Rosenfeld CR, Battaglia FC, *et al.* Effect of estrogens on the uterine blood flow of oophorectomized ewes. *Am J Obstet Gynecol* 1973; 115:1045–52

9. Volterrani M, Rosano GMC, Clark AL, *et al.* Haemodynamic effects of acute administration of estradiol-17β. *Am J Med* 1995;99:119–122 (Abstract)

10. Rosano GMC, Sarrel PM, Poole-Wilson PA, *et al.* Beneficial effect of estrogen on exercise-induced myocardial ischemia in women with coronary artery disease. *Lancet* 1993;342:133–6

11. Holdright DR, Sullivan AK, Wright CA, *et al.* Acute effect of oestrogen replacement therapy on treadmill performance in post-menopausal women with coronary artery disease. *Eur Heart J* 1994;15:546 (Abstract)

12. Al-Khalili F, Schenck-Gustafsson K, Eksborg S, *et al.* Acute administration of sublingual 2 mg 17 beta estradiol shows no effect on exercise-induced coronary ischemia in post-menopausal women with stable angina pectoris. *Eur Heart J* 1996;17(Suppl) (Abstract)

13. Cobbe SM, Poole-Wilson PA. Continuous coronary sinus and arterial pH monitoring during pacing-induced ischemia in coronary artery disease. *Br Heart J* 1982;47:369–74

14. Cobbe SM, Parker DJ, Poole-Wilson PA. Tissue and coronary venous pH in ischemic canine myocardium. *Clin Cardiol* 1982;5:153–6

15. Cobbe SM, Poole-Wilson PA. Catheter tip pH electrodes for continuous intravascular recording. *J Med Eng Technol* 1980;4:122–4

16. Rosano GMC, Mendes Caixeta A, Arie S, *et al.* Acute anti ischemic effect of estradiol 17 beta in menopausal women with coronary artery disease. *J Am Coll Cardiol* 1996;27:2(Suppl A) (Abstract)

17. Collins P, Rosano GMC, Sarrel PM, *et al.* 17β-estradiol attenuates acetylcholine-induced coronary arterial constriction in women but not in men with coronary heart disease. *Circulation* 1995;92:24–30

18. Caulin-Glaser TL, Sessa W, Sarrel PM, *et al.* Estradiol stimulates NO production via transcriptional and non-transcriptional pathways. *Circulation* 1995;90:I-30(Abstract)

19. Rosano GMC, Lopez Hidalgo M, Arie S, *et al.* Acute effect of 17 beta estradiol upon coronary artery reactivity in menopausal women with coronary artery disease. *Eur Heart J* 1996; 17 (Suppl) (Abstract)

20. Collins P, Shay J, Jiang C, *et al.* Nitric oxide accounts for dose-dependent oestrogen-mediated coronary relaxation following acute oestrogen withdrawal. *Circulation* 1994;90: 1964–8

21. Furchgott RF, Zawadzki JV. The obligatory role of endothelial cells in the relaxation of arterial smooth muscle by acetylcholine. *Nature (London)* 1980;288:373–6

22. Williams JK, Adams MR, Klopfenstein HS. Oestrogen modulates responses of atherosclerotic coronary arteries. *Circulation* 1990;81:1680–87

23. Gilligan DM, Quyumi AA, Cannon RO III. Effects of physiological levels of oestrogen on coronary vasomotor function in postmenopausal women. *Circulation* 1994;89:2545–51

24. Ball P, Knuppen R, Bruer H. Interactions between oestrogens and catecholamines: III. Studies on the methylation of catechol oestrogens, catecholamines, and other catechols by the catechol-*o*-methyltransferase of human liver. *J Clin Endocrinol* 1972;34:736–46

25. Hamlet MA, Rorie DK, Tyce GM. Effects of estradiol on release and disposition of norepinephrine from nerve endings. *Am J Physiol* 1980;239:H450–H456

26. Sarrel PM. Ovarian hormones and the circulation. *Maturitas* 1990;12:287–98

27. Pfaff DW. Impact of oestrogens on hypothalamic nerve cells: ultrastructural, chemical and electrical effects. *Recent Prog Horm Res* 1983;39:127–79

28. Kronenberg F, Cote LJ, Linkie DM, *et al.* Menopausal hot flashes: thermo-regulatory, cardiovascular, and circulating catecholamine and LH changes. *Maturitas* 1984;6:31–43

29. Krinenberg F. Hot flashes: epidemiology and physiology. *Ann NY Acad Sci* 1990;592:52–86

30. Davidson L, Rouse IL, Vandongen R, *et al.* Plasma noradrenaline and its relationship to plasma oestradiol in normal women during the menstrual cycle. *Clin Exp Pharmacol Physiol* 1985;12:489–93

31. Rosano GMC, Leonardo F, Ponikowski P, *et al.* Estrogen replacement therapy normalizes the autonomic control of the cardiovascular system in menopausal women. *J Am Coll Cardiol* 1996;27:2 (Suppl A) (Abstract)

Coronary artery disease in postmenopausal women: 10 years' experience in a coronary care unit

10

J. Lopo Tuna, A.L. Bordalo-Sá, A.L. Santos, L. Neves, M. Melo, C. Ribeiro and J.T. Soares-Costa

An increasing interest in the treatment and health care of women suffering from coronary artery disease (CAD) has occurred over recent years. Traditionally there has been an under-investigation of CAD in women. Therapeutic interventional studies that have established the advantages of aspirin or drugs producing hypolipidemia in secondary prevention of CAD have been performed mostly, if not exclusively, in men[1]. Similarly, survival studies after coronary revascularization surgery in the 1970s were performed only in male patients[2]. However, CAD has a significant incidence in women and is an important cause of mortality, particularly in the elderly. American statistics show that, after the age of 60 years, CAD is the main cause of death in women[3]. In the USA the absolute number of annual deaths from acute myocardial infarction (AMI) in ages ≥ 65 years is similar in both genders (440 000 in males and 374 000 in females)[3].

In a paper published in 1982[4], the Coronary Care Unit of Santa Maria Hospital, in Lisbon, highlighted the importance of AMI in women, presenting the data on 300 women admitted with AMI between the years of 1973 and 1980. The dramatic advances in the fields of diagnosis and therapy that have occurred since then, and the possibility of eventual epidemiological changes, justify an update of these historical findings.

In the present paper we review the data concerning female patients with AMI admitted to our Coronary Care Unit (CCU) during a 10-year period, from 1986 to 1995; we compare them with data on male patients admitted during the same period and with the group of patients studied during the 1970s.

PATIENTS AND METHODS

The information in the files of the CCU of Santa Maria Hospital dates from 1985[5-7]. This information system automatically generates a database which is filled from the day of admission, being brought up to date daily during the stay of the patients in the department and closed on the day of discharge, generating a computerized report that is given to the patient for conveyance to their physician. The data initially collected can be corrected through the introduction of new data (for example: results of examinations unknown when the patient is discharged). This core system is connected to another database which includes the findings of the follow-up of patients after hospital discharge.

Currently the database includes the records of 5200 patients, perhaps being considered one of the largest databases in the world concerning patients suffering from CAD treated by the same medical group with standardized inclusion criteria and diagnosis.

To perform the present study, we retrieved from the database the values of the variables referring to patients with the diagnosis of AMI. The diagnostic criteria were in accordance with the guidelines of the World Health Organization (WHO)[8] and were approved in Portugal by the Portuguese Society of Cardiology[9].

From the total number of 2439 patients admitted between 1986 and 1995, we studied the following parameters: gender, age and inhospital mortality (general and in both genders).

In a more restricted group of patients, admitted more recently, during a 3-year period between 1993 and 1995, from a total number of 655 patients, we looked for the number of patients submitted to fibrinolytic therapy, the number of patients admitted up to 6 h from onset of the clinical picture of AMI and the prevalence of some classical risk factors for CAD, namely arterial hypertension, dyslipidemia, smoking and diabetes mellitus. The classification was based on data from the anamnesis obtained during the admission. Information given by patients' relatives and data on treatment were of some use.

In the absence of a specific inquiry, and since there is no epidemiological study on this topic in our country, 50 years old was considered as the age of menopause in Portugal.

Control group: retrospective study (1973–80)

The results of the present study were compared to those of the retrospective study made in our CCU, involving the review of 300 clinical case reports of women consecutively admitted between 1973 and 1980, which was published in 1982[4]. In this study the mean age of the patients was 67 ± 10 years, with a variation interval between 41 and 90 years old. Out of the 300 patients, 281 were > 50 years old (94%) (Table 1). During the hospital stay, 87 patients died (hospital mortality of 29% in women).

Considering the mortality rate by decade of life, we observed a progressive increase in every decade: 11% before 51 years old, 22% in the age group of 51–60, 26% in the age group of 61–70 and 35% in patients older than 70.

Statistical analysis

The χ^2 2×2 test with the Yates correction was used in the comparison of proportions. A value of $p < 0.05$ was considered as statistically significant.

Table 1 Mortality by age group in 300 women admitted with acute myocardial infarction in the 1970s (from reference 4)

Age group (years)	Number	Deaths	%
41–50	19	2	11
51–60	41	9	22
61–70	111	31	28
71–80	107	37	35
81–90	22	8	37
Total	300	87	29

RESULTS

Distribution of the cases of acute myocardial infarction according to sex and age

A total of 2439 patients with the diagnosis of AMI were admitted to our CCU during the time interval between 1986 and 1995: 521 females (F) and 1198 males (M), corresponding to a M:F ratio of 3.5:1 (Figure 1). In accordance with the age groups, the M:F ratio was very different: 336 men and 30 women younger than 50 years old were admitted, representing a M:F ratio of 11:1. On the other hand, 1582 men and 491 women older than 50 years were admitted, providing a M:F ratio of 3:1 (Figure 2). The postmenopausal M:F ratio decreased as the age increased: 7:1 in the sixth decade, 3:1 in the seventh decade and 1.8:1 in the elderly ≥ 70 years (Figure 1).

A review of 30 case reports of women less than 50 years old was carried out. There was reference to surgical menopause in one case and to physiological menopause in three more cases, in which menopause occurred during the second half of the fifth decade, less than 12 months before the date of AMI. Considering all 521 women studied, 80% were older than 60 years and 46% were older than 70 years.

Mortality

A total of 355 patients died, which corresponds to a general mortality of 14.5%. The mortality was influenced by the age of

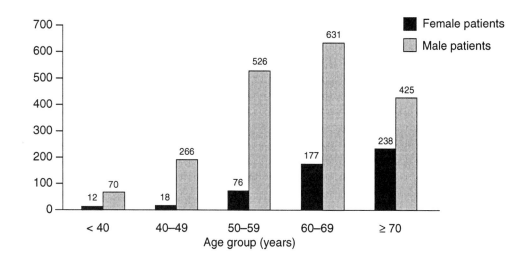

Figure 1 Distribution of the cases of acute myocardial infarction according to sex and age

the patients. Only 13 out of 366 patients younger than 50 years died (3.5%) vs. 342 out of 2073 patients with ages of 50 years or more (16.5%) (Figure 3). Death occurred in 135 out of 521 women (25.9%) and 220 out of 1198 men (12.0%) ($p < 0.001$).

In Figure 4 we show the percentage distribution of mortality by sex and age groups. There was a progressive growth of mortality as age increased in both genders: until the age of 59 the mortality was almost equal in both genders, but at greater ages

there was a higher increase in mortality in female patients. Mortality was 25% in women vs. 12% in men ($p < 0.001$) in the seventh decade and 36% in women vs. 24% in men ($p < 0.005$) in patients older than 70 years.

Comparing this group of patients to the control group of the retrospective study of the 1970s, the global mortality in women decreased from 29% to 25.9% (p NS). The mortality by decade of life was similar: in patients older than 70 years, 36% in the control group and 36% in the current study;

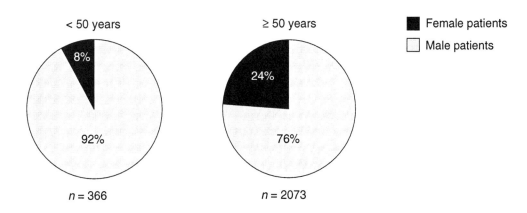

Figure 2 Relationship of women : men in cases of acute myocardial infarction

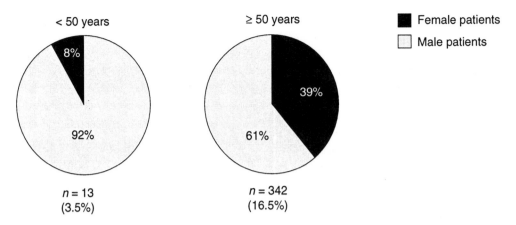

Figure 3 Relationship of women : men in mortality from acute myocardial infarction. *n*, number of patients who died

28% and 25%, respectively, between 60 and 69 years old (*p* NS); 22% and 7%, respectively, between 50 and 59 years (*p* < 0.05); and in patients younger than 50 years the mortality was 11% in the group of patients of the 1970 study vs. 3.3% in the current study (*p* NS).

Thrombolytic therapy

During the 3-year period between 1993 and 1995, 655 patients suffering from AMI were admitted to the CCU: 147 women and 508 men. Thrombolytic therapy was performed in 33 women (23%) and 141 men (28%) (*p* NS). Arrival at the CCU in sufficient time to perform thrombolytic therapy, that is to say during the first 6 h from the onset of the clinical picture of AMI, occurred in 52 women (35%) and in 199 men (39%).

Risk factors

In the same group of patients admitted between 1993 and 1995 we analyzed the

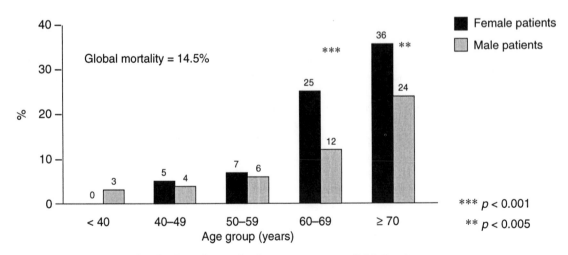

Figure 4 Sex and age distribution of mortality from acute myocardial infarction

presence of some classical risk factors for CAD – arterial hypertension, dyslipidemia, diabetes mellitus and smoking.

Arterial hypertension was significantly more prevalent in women admitted with AMI than in men (66% vs. 46%, respectively; $p < 0.001$). Diabetes mellitus was significantly more prevalent in women than in men (31% vs. 20%, respectively, $p < 0.01$). A previous history of dyslipidemia was more frequent in women than in men, although the difference was not statistically significant (24% vs. 19%, respectively; p NS). On the other hand, smoking was a risk factor significantly less frequent in women than in men (11% vs. 44%, respectively, $p < 0.001$).

DISCUSSION

The results of this study confirm the assertion that CAD, under its form of AMI, occurs quite rarely in premenopausal women. Out of the total cases of AMI in women, AMI was observed in women younger than 50 years old (6%) in only 30 cases and at least four of these cases occurred in menopausal women. The occurrence of AMI before the age of 60 was also not frequent: only 76 cases were seen between 50 and 59 years old (14%), i.e. 80% of the AMI in women occurred after the age of 60, about 10 years after the age of physiological menopause. This is not a surprising fact, as menopause only marks a moment in the gradual weakening of ovarian function which is prolonged for a period that can last for about 10 years[10]. In contrast, there is a sudden increase of the risk for CAD in women submitted to surgical menopause with bilateral ovariectomy and not submitted to hormonal replacement therapy (HRT), this risk being approximately 2.2 times greater than that in premenopausal women of the same age[3].

The relationship between estrogen deficiency and the risk of CAD is well established[11]. Part of the protection given by estrogen (perhaps 50%) depends on the beneficial effect of estrogen on circulating lipoproteins, particularly on the elevation of high-density lipoprotein (HDL)-cholesterol. Estrogen also lowers the low-density lipoprotein (LDL)-cholesterol and increases triglyceridemia, but triglyceride elevation has no clinical importance[12]. Hormonal replacement therapy in postmenopausal women is supported by a large number of studies that point to a reduction of 44% in the risk for CAD in treated women[13].

During the 10-year period of our study, mortality in women was significantly higher than in men (26% vs. 12%, respectively; $p < 0.001$). But the excess in mortality was not independent of age; on the contrary it appeared only in the older age groups, from 60 to 69 years and more than 70 years. Until the age of 60, mortality was always very low and similar in both sexes (Figure 4). It is interesting to make the comparison of mortality occurring in our CCU in female patients by decade of life between the years 1973–80 (control group) and 1986–95 (present study). The global mortality decreased in a nonsignificant way from 29% to 26%. It was similar in patients older than 70 years, slightly decreased between 60 and 69 years (28% to 25%), a significant decrease being seen in the younger groups of patients, from 22% to 7% ($p < 0.05$) between 50 and 59 years old and from 10% to 3% (p NS) in patients younger than 50 years old.

In highly selected populations, as was the case of the patients that we admitted in a reference CCU of a central hospital with access to urgent cardiac surgery, it is generally recognized that it is of small importance to speak of the mortality from AMI. The population of the admitted patients presents an important percentage of complicated cases, distorting, for the worse, the mortality. While during the 1970s it was quite normal to transfer patients to the coronary care units who were initially admitted to district hospitals on account of rhythmic complications, nowadays the main reasons for this kind of transfer are mechanical complications. This is the reason why the limited reduction of mortality observed in a 15-year interval does not mean that the dramatic advances in therapy achieved in recent years had no repercussion on a better short-term prognosis for our patients. The results seem to indicate that it is easier to detect those advantages in younger patients, namely under the age of 60.

Another explanation is that we are not giving to women the same opportunities of treatment we are giving to men. In this context the Yentl syndrome is well known[14] (named after the heroine of the Boris Isaac Singer novel, a Jewish woman who had to be disguised as a man in order to proceed with her studies). The problem was raised by a subgroup analysis of the Survival and Ventricular Enlargement (SAVE) study[15] in which, after an acute myocardial infarction, the treatments received by men and women were compared. Women presented angina before AMI in the same proportion to men, but they had half the probability of being submitted to cardiac catheterization and to coronary bypass heart surgery. The analysis of this phenomenon was not part of the objectives of the present study, which did not evaluate the access to cardiac catheterization and revascularization therapy after AMI, but we had the opportunity of observing the access to another kind of therapy, whose difference between both sexes, discriminating against women, has been another mentioned cause for the higher mortality from AMI in women. We are referring to fibrinolytic therapy. Many authors have written that thrombolytic therapy is less frequently used in women because they show more contraindications than men, one of them being their more advanced age and their later arrival in the hospital, which could be explained by a less evocative clinical picture with a high incidence of atypical symptoms. Women have a higher risk of hemorrhagic stroke[16]. Sexual discrimination in the access to fibrinolytic therapy is not confirmed in our CCU. This kind of treatment was lower in women than in men (23% vs. 28%, respectively), but the difference was not statistically significant.

The recognized higher frequency of atypical cases in women was not reflected in a later arrival of the patients to the hospital. Of the women, 35% vs. 39% of the men were admitted to our CCU within the first 6 h of evolution of the clinical picture of AMI.

It is known that the presence of risk factors in the history of patients suffering from AMI is higher in women than in men. The data from our department reveal that, of the classical risk factors, only smoking was more prevalent in men (44% in men and 11% in women; $p < 0.001$), explained by cultural reasons. The female patients admitted to our hospital are generally elderly women who did not smoke during their youth. As time goes by, habits are changing, and it is expected that this percentage difference between women and men will decrease progressively in the future as a consequence of the trend to equalization of the smoking habits of both sexes. Even in the USA, where the reduction of tobacco consumption is a fact, the decreasing rate of smoking is lower in women than in men[3]. This might be caused by some kind of advertisements especially directed towards women, passing the message that smoking is a way of getting thin, as well as by the promotion of 'light' cigarettes with low tar, nicotine and carbon monoxide rates. Epidemiological data indicate, however, that 'light' cigarette smokers are not at lower risk of CAD than 'normal' cigarette consumers[17].

The prevalence of a previous history of hypercholesterolemia was higher in women than in men, although the difference was not statistically significant (24% vs. 19%, respectively). We all know that the diagnosis of hypercholesterolemia from the anamnesis of patients admitted with AMI is a difficult one. Hypolipemiant therapy is not very much diffused among our patients so this kind of medication is not a useful diagnostic criterion. On the other hand, during the acute phase of myocardial infarction, and particularly after the first 24 h, there was a decrease in serum lipid levels lasting for a period of 2–3 months. This is the reason that the determinations of the serum lipid levels during the stay in hospital were significantly different from the baseline values. The true prevalence of dyslipidemia in patients suffering from AMI is probably higher than the percentage calculated on the basis of patient anamnesis, and this is likely to be true for both women and men.

It is questionable whether the extrapolation is feasible to women of the results of some studies in men which show that the decrease in serum cholesterol levels is associated with a reduction in the of risk of CAD. The antioxidant effects of estrogen interfere with the lipid profile, so LDL-cholesterol may not be as strong a predicting risk factor in women as in men. Extrapolation of the LDL-cholesterol from the total cholesterol levels is also not possible, because HDL-cholesterol is higher in women than in men and so its contribution to the total cholesterol value is higher[18]. HDL-cholesterol is a stronger risk predictor in women than in men[19]. Similarly, triglycerides, which have only a weak association with risk for CAD in men, are a stronger risk index in women according to the Framingham Study[20].

Until recently, there was a great difference in recruitment of men and women in the trials of hypolipemiant drugs for secondary prevention of CAD. For 1000 men only 400 women were recruited[3]. However, these small numbers were enough to suggest that the efficacy of this kind of treatment was similar in both sexes. The results of some recent trials, such as the 4S which involved 1445 men and 827 women (more than double the number of recruited women than in all the previous secondary prevention studies), have shown, probably definitively, that the same degree of reduction of cholesterolemia in men and women is accompanied by the same degree of reduction of mortality caused by CAD in both sexes. In the 4S study there was a 35% reduction of the risk for major coronary events in treated women[21].

The prevalence of arterial hypertension was significantly higher in female patients than in men (66% vs. 46%, respectively; $p < 0.001$). In contrast to the interventional studies on lipids for the secondary prevention of CAD, in a meta-analysis of the controlled studies with pharmacological intervention in patients with slight to moderate hypertension and CAD, involving 37 000 subjects, 47% of the patients included[22] were women. There were obvious and important benefits in both sexes. Elderly women represent a special focus. Systolic arterial hypertension resulting from loss of elasticity of the arterial wall is more prevalent in women than in men. It is admitted that systolic arterial hypertension affects approximately 30% of women older than 65[23]. In the Systolic Hypertension in the Elderly Program, in which women represented 57% of the studied population, the anti-hypertensive treatment resulted in a 36% reduction in strokes and 25% reduction in cases of CAD[24].

Diabetes mellitus is a particularly important risk factor in women. There is evidence that the protection that women have against atherosclerosis is almost completely lost in the presence of diabetes. Diabetic men and women have approximately the same risk for CAD in every age group[25]. The mortality rates from CAD in diabetic women are three to seven times higher than in non-diabetic women. In diabetic men mortality rates from CAD are two to four times higher than in non-diabetic men[26]. The higher risk associated with diabetes in women seems to be a function of their higher survival in the absence of diabetes: the interaction between diabetes, sex and coronary risk is not due to higher mortality rates for CAD in diabetic women in relation to diabetic men, but to a lower rate of mortality in non-diabetic women in relation to non-diabetic men. It has been suggested that the serum levels of HDL-cholesterol are lower in diabetic women than in diabetic men, which could explain their higher risk for CAD[27]. Diabetes increases the known risk factor effects and can block the connection to estrogen, decreasing the protection against CAD given by the endogenous estrogen in premenopausal woman. In the population of our study the previous history of diabetes mellitus was significantly more frequent in women than in men (31% vs. 20%, respectively; $p < 0.01$).

The higher prevalence of risk factors for CAD among women in comparison to men indicates that women are more protected. Women suffering an AMI tend to be older than men and to have more associated diseases. This finding of our study confirms similar observations in studies performed in other countries.

In conclusion, the risk of AMI is very low in premenopausal women. As age increases there is a reduction of the M:F ratio in the incidence of AMI, as seen in our study, from 11:1 in people < 50 years to 1.8:1 in people ≥ 70 years old. The risk of death increases progressively with age in both sexes, but while it is similar in men and women until the age of 60, in older people the mortality is significantly higher in women. Women, besides being older than men when they suffer an AMI, also have a higher prevalence of risk factors for CAD, namely arterial hypertension, diabetes mellitus and dyslipidemia.

ACKNOWLEDGEMENT

We wish to thank Ms Honorina Correia for the preparation of the manuscript.

References

1. La Rosa JC, Hunninghake D, Bush D, *et al.* The cholesterol facts: a summary of the evidence relating dietary fats, serum cholesterol and coronary heart disease: a joint statement by the American Heart Association and the National Heart, Lung, and Blood Institute. *Circulation* 1990;81:1721–33

2. Alderman EL, Bourassa MG, Cohen LS, *et al.* Ten-year follow-up of survival and myocardial infarction in the randomized Coronary Artery Surgery Study. *Circulation* 1990;82:1629–46

3. Rich-Edwards JW, Manson JE, Hennekens CH, *et al.* The primary prevention of coronary heart disease in women. *N Engl J Med* 1995;332:1758–66

4. Ferreira RJ, Rebelo VJ, Bordalo ADB, *et al.* Perfil clínico do enfarte do miocárdico no sexo feminino. *Rev Port Cardiol* 1982;2:33–9

5. Laureano Santos A, Roxo Covas A, Silva CA, *et al.* Automatic information system for a coronary care unit. In *Computers in Cardiology.* Los Angeles: IEEE Computer Society, 1987:641–3

6. Laureano Santos A. O arquivo informatizado da UTIC-Arsénio Cordeiro. In Ribeiro C, Tuna JL, eds. *Cuidados Intensivos para Doentes das Coronárias.* Lisbon: Neo-Farma-Cêutica 1988:21–7

7. Laureano Santos A. Um sistema de informação automatizado para unidades coronárias. Sua aplicação na avaliação do prognóstico hospitalar do enfarte do miocárdio. Faculdade de Medicina de Lisboa. Lisbon: Authors' edition 1991:199

8. Joint International Society and Federation of Cardiology/World Health Organization Task Force on Standardization of Clinical Nomenclature. Nomenclature and criteria for diagnosis of ischemic heart disease. *Circulation* 1979; 59:607–9

9. Araújo A, Calçada Correia L, Morais I, *et al.* Nomenclatura da doença cardíaca isquémica 1ª Reunião Nacional sobre Recomendações, Competências e Consensos em Cardiologia. *Rev Port Cardiol* 1989;8(Suppl 2):255–9

10. Stampfer MJ, Colditz GA, Willett WC. Menopause and heart disease: a review. *Ann NY Acad Sci* 1990;592:193–203

11. Kannel WB, Gordon T, eds. Probability of developing certain cardiovascular diseases in eight years at specified values of some characteristics. *Framingham Study, Epidemiological Investigation of Cardiovascular Disease.* Rockville, MD: DHEW Publication (NIH), 1973:74–618 (Section 28)

12. Walsh BW, Schiff I, Rosner B, *et al.* Effects of postmenopausal estrogen replacement on the concentrations and metabolism of lipoproteins. *N Engl J Med* 1991;325:1196–204

13. Stampfer MJ, Colditz GA. Estrogen replacement therapy and coronary heart disease: quantitative assessment of the epidemiologic evidence. *Prev Med* 1991;20:47–63

14. Healy AB. The Yentl syndrome. *N Engl J Med* 1991;325:274–6

15. Steingart RM, Packer MP, Hamm P, *et al.* Sex differences in the management of coronary artery disease. *N Engl J Med* 1991;325:226–30

16. Lincoff AM, Califf RM, Ellis SG, *et al.* JD, for the Thrombolysis and Angioplasty in Myocardial Infarction Study Group. Thrombolysis therapy for women with myocardial infarction: is there a gender gap? *J Am Coll Cardiol* 1993;22:1780–7

17. Palmer JR, Rosenberg L, Shapiro S. 'Low yield' cigarettes and the risk of nonfatal myocardial infarction in women. *N Engl J Med* 1989;320:1569–73

18. LaRosa LC. Dyslipoproteinemia in women and the elderly. *Med Clin North Am* 1994;78:163–80

19. Bush TL, Fried LP, Barrett-Connor E. Cholesterol, lipoproteins, and coronary heart disease in women. *Clin Chem* 1988;34:B60

20. Castelli WP. The triglyceride issue: a view from Framingham. *Am Heart J* 1986;112:432–7.

21. Scandinavian Simvastatin Study Group. Randomised trial of cholesterol lowering in 4444 patients with coronary heart disease: The Scandinavian Simvastatin Survival Study (4S). *Lancet* 1994;334:1383–9

22. Collins R, Peto R, MacMahon S, *et al.* Blood pressure, stroke and coronary heart disease. 2. Short-term reductions in blood pressure: overview of randomized drug trials in their epidemiological context. *Lancet* 1990;335:827–38

23. Saltzberg S, Stroh JA, Frishman WH. Isolated systolic hypertension in the elderly: pathophysiology and treatment. *Med Clin North Am* 1988;72:523–47

24. SHEP Cooperative Research Group. Prevention of stroke by antihypertensive drug treatment in older persons with isolated systolic hypertension: final results of the Systolic Hypertension in the Elderly Program (SHEP). *J Am Med Assoc* 1991;265:3255–64

25. Krolewski AS, Warram JE, Valsania P, *et al.* Evolving natural history of coronary artery disease in diabetes mellitus. *Am J Med* 1991;90 (Suppl 2A):2A-56S

26. Pan WH, Cedres LB, Liu K, *et al.* Relationship of clinical diabetes and asymptomatic hyperglycemia to risk of coronary heart disease mortality in men and women. *Am J Epidemiol* 1986;123:504–16

27. Walden CE, Knopp RH, Wahl PW, *et al.* Sex differences in the effect of diabetes mellitus on lipoprotein triglyceride and cholesterol concentrations. *N Engl J Med* 1984;311:953–9

Lipid changes induced by HRT administered by different routes

11

M. Birkhäuser and W. Haenggi

INTRODUCTION

Cardiovascular diseases are today among the leading causes of death in males and females. After menopause, the female risk for cardiovascular accidents approaches the male risk. At the age of 65 years, death is due to a coronaropathy in one out of three women. In Europe, the US and Australia, about 10 times more women are dying from coronary diseases than from breast cancer, and significantly more women succumb to coronaropathies than to cerebrovascular diseases, infections, gastrointestinal affections, respiratory diseases or diabetes mellitus and its complications (Vital statistics of the United States, II; NIH-79-1102). The exponential increase of cardiovascular mortality in women after menopause points to an important physiological role of estrogens for the integrity of the cardiovascular system[1-3].

Cardiovascular diseases are responsible for 54% of all deaths secondary to coronary pathologies. Although most patients fear dying from cancer, many more people are victims of cardiovascular diseases, cerebrovascular accidents, infections, gastrointestinal or pulmonary diseases, and diabetes mellitus and its consequences than of carcinomas. It is well known that the incidence of cardiovascular disease differs significantly between males and females before the age of 50 years[4]. Up to that age, the relative risk of dying from a coronary heart disease is in males 2.24 ± 0.08 times greater than in women. Because, after menopause, the female risk progressively approaches the male risk, gynecological endocrinologists became increasingly interested in cardiovascular diseases. Their

hypothesis was that this difference might be explained by the different profile of sex steroids and has been confirmed by the results of several large epidemiological studies in retirement communities in the USA[5,6]. These studies have demonstrated that estrogen replacement therapy can reduce the risk of dying from a cardiovascular disease by approximately 50%. Inversely, estrogen deficiency has been shown to be the main risk factor for cardiovascular diseases in women[7,8].

However, another significant difference between the sexes has to be considered. About 50% of all women suffering from symptoms compatible with angina pectoris have intact arteries at coronary angiography[9], whereas in males the percentage of subjects having healthy coronaries is only 10%. This syndrome (angina pectoris in the presence of normal coronaries) is caused by arterial spasms and has been named 'syndrome X'[10-12]. It is characterized by electrocardiographic alterations suspicious of ischemia during effort, with normal coronaries. Syndrome X can usually be treated successfully by the administration of estrogens. Estrogens modulate also the vasomotor response of atherosclerotic coronary arteries.

An important clinical difference between the sexes known since 1901[13] is the fact that women presenting identically serious objective alterations of the coronaries suffer quite frequently from lighter subjective symptoms[14]. Therefore, the cardiovascular disease is often diagnosed later than in the male and some diagnostic tools, e.g. coronary angiography, are used more often in males than in women. Clinical data show, too, that women suffering from acute myocardial infarction are on average 7–8 years older than men with a first heart attack. Furthermore, there are clinical differences in the evolution of an acute coronary accident. Women suffering from diagnosed coronary disease have a higher mortality rate than males. After a first myocardial infarction, 39% of the women concerned will die compared to only 31% of the males. Today, there are serious indications that secondary prevention by estrogens can significantly ameliorate the unfavorable prognosis for the outcome after a heart attack in women. However, additional data are needed to confirm these highly interesting observations[9,15–17].

What is the mechanism through which insufficient secretion of estrogens has a negative effect and normal secretion of estrogens has a protective effect on the vascular wall? It is believed that two independent mechanisms participate in this vascular action:

(1) Direct estrogen action at the arterial wall[18–23]. This effect is presented by another paper in these proceedings;

(2) Indirect estrogen action via alterations of the lipid profile[24–30]. This indirect effect is the main subject of the present review.

The importance of these two mechanisms is variable. It is agreed that the direct estrogenic action at the endothelium of the arterial wall is responsible for 70–80% of the protective estrogen activity. In contrast, the indirect action through a change of the lipid profile adds 20–30% to cardioprotection.

THE PATHOPHYSIOLOGICAL IMPORTANCE OF DIFFERENT LIPIDS

Atherogenic lipoproteins

By definition, the density of very low-density lipoproteins (VLDL) is less than 1.006 g/ml. VLDL are formed by the secretion of endogenously synthesized triglycerides together with cholesterol and phos-

pholipids. Each VLDL particle contains a protein molecule, apolipoprotein (apo)-B proteins and different amounts of lipids combined with smaller proteins, apo-E and apo-C. The triglycerides contained within the VLDL are hydrolyzed in the periphery enzymatically by liapses. During this process, the surface lipids of the VLDL complexes are released. These lipids can be transferred to high-density lipoproteins (HDL). The remnants of VLDL are eliminated by the liver. Most probably, low-density lipoprotein (LDL) receptors and proteins similar to LDL receptors participate in this process. Exogenous lipids are treated similarly to endogenous triglycerides. If small VLDL particles remain for a longer period within the circulation, intermediate-density lipoproteins (IDL, density 1.006–1.019 g/ml) and finally LDL (density 1.019–1.063 g/ml) can be formed through the transfer of certain VLDL residues and by the combination with other cholesterol particles. The most important components of LDL particles are apo-B proteins and cholesterol esters. In the peripheral circulation, the most important part of cholesterol is formed by LDL particles. VLDL, IDL and LDL are heterogeneous and are formed by several subpopulations characterized by different size, density and composition. The main parts of IDL and LDL are bound by hepatic LDL receptors and eliminated from the circulation. Another mechanism to retain LDL within the tissue is the uptake by macrophages. This mechanism is considered to be the critical step within the arterial wall that initiates the process of atherosclerosis and that continues progressively to the smooth muscle cells. It is still unknown whether the oxidation of lipids leads to other substances which also participate in the formation of atherosclerosis by initiating the proliferation of cellular elements and by changing the function of thrombocytes. Therefore, LDL belong, like triglycerides, to the 'unfavorable' lipids, whereas HDL (see below) belong to the 'favorable' ones.

High-density lipoproteins

HDL are as heterogeneous as LDL lipoproteins are. They are formed by several lipids and proteins. Their metabolic pattern, too, is variable. Typically, HDL particles contain apolipoproteins type A1 originating from the liver and from the intestinal region. A smaller part of HDL particles contains apolipoproteins type A2, type C and type E. It is generally accepted that the greatest part of HDL particles is formed from precursors poor in lipids which take up additional lipids and are transformed during their presence within the circulation in different ways. HDL are not only formed by the metabolism of apo-B complexes, but also through the direct uptake of cellular lipids, particularly non-esterified cholesterol. Apo-A1 activates a specific enzyme for the esterification of non-esterified cholesterol and enables the progressive uptake of cholesterol and apo-proteins. The smaller and denser subclasses of HDL are called HDL-3 and the larger HDL particles HDL-2. Large HDL-2 molecules are more frequent in women than in men and correlate with the plasma HDL-cholesterol concentrations.

HDL is able to transport cholesterol from the peripheral tissues to the liver. This capacity leads to the hypothesis that HDL has an anti-atherogenic potency in carrying cholesterol from the blood vessels to the liver. However, other factors could also participate in the favorable effect of HDL on the risk for atherosclerosis. For instance, high HDL levels could point at lower plasma levels or a shorter presence within the plasma of some small and potentially atherogenic particles. HDL could also reduce the accumulation of lipid peroxidases within the LDL complexes. Data from experiments done in animals suggest that an increased apo-A1 production reduces atherogenesis.

Lipoprotein (a)

Lipoprotein (a) (Lp (a)) contains apolipoprotein B-100 complexes together with another large protein, apolipoprotein (a),

which greatly resembles plasminogen. The plasma concentrations of Lp (a) are highly variable among the normal healthy population and are probably under direct and constant genetic control. Epidemiological studies show a strong correlation between the levels of Lp (a) and the risk for coronary pathology. Apo (a) has been found directly within arterial lesions. The exact mechanism through which Lp (a) is involved in atherogenesis is not yet known, but the fibrinolytic system could participate to a large extent.

THE INFLUENCE OF PERORAL AND TRANSDERMAL ESTROGEN ON THE LIPID PATTERN

Triglycerides and VLDL

In the peroral route of administration, the levels of triglycerides and VLDL increase proportionally to the dosage of the estrogen given[27-32]. This increase is absent in transdermal administration[31,33]. Perorally administered estrogens have been show to increase the triglyceride levels by a higher hepatic production rate and to stimulate the secretion of VLDL-apo-protein 100. In contrast, in transdermal estrogen administration, triglyceride levels remain within the normal range, as illustrated by our own data[34] (Table 1). In the peroral treatment group, triglycerides increased significantly at 6 and 12 months compared to baseline, and VLDL-cholesterol only at 12 months. Both patterns have to be considered as unfavorable. In the transdermal treatment group, this unwanted rise of the triglyceride levels was not observed. When estrogens were administered transdermally, there was also no change in the plasma levels of VLDL-cholesterol, rich in triglycerides. VLDL is kown to correlate directly with triglyceride levels.

Total cholesterol and LDL-cholesterol

Total cholesterol and LDL-cholesterol both decrease during hormonal substitution[27-31]. Conjugated equine estrogens, micronized

17β-estradiol and 17β-estradiol valerate given perorally significantly decrease the levels of LDL and increase, also significantly, the levels of HDL. In peroral administration, the LDL changes are proportional to the amount of estrogens administered[32]. In the literature, the LDL changes induced by 0.625 mg of conjugated estrogens or 2 mg of estradiol valerate are reported to vary between 11 and 15%. Our own data (Table 1) show a significant LDL decrease for the transdermal administration of 17β-estradiol (50 μg/day). However, the mechanism of the transdermally induced LDL decrease is not clear.

In our study[34], a significant decrease of total cholesterol was observed only in the transdermal group at 6 and at 12 months, compared to baseline. At 12 months, the decrease was 5% ($p < 0.05$). Epidemiological data show that a decrease in total cholesterol by 1% reduces the risk of a new cardiovascular accident by 2%.

It is interesting to note a significant decrease of LDL-cholesterol at 6 and 12 months, not only in the peroral but also in the transdermal treatment group. This change has to be considered as favorable.

The decrease of the atherogenic LDL is, in both treatment groups, the consequence of an estrogen-induced increase of the synthesis of LDL receptors. Following our data, this mechanism has to function significantly not only in the peroral, but also in the transdermal route of administration. This effect might not have been found by other research groups because, in these studies, other progestagens have been used, such as medroxyprogesterone acetate. Apolipoprotein-B, the main apolipoprotein of LDL (not listed in Table 1) increased in our study in parallel to LDL. At 12 months, the difference in apo-B was highly significant between the control group and the treatement groups. Again, the prognostic value is favorable in the treated population.

HDL-cholesterol

The administration of estrogens increases HDL-cholesterol, particularly the levels of the HDL-2 fraction[35]. When 0.625 mg conjugated estrogens corresponding to 2 mg 17β-estradiol was administered, the average HDL rise reached 10–15%. Dose dependency is less pronounced in the changes of HDL than of LDL.

A high peroral estrogen dosage especially stimulates the production rate of HDL apo-A1. In addition, estrogen substitution significantly reduces the activity of hepatic lipase and decreases the HDL clearance. This mechanism results most probably in a particularly pronounced elevation of the HDL-2 subclasses. In the control group, our data show a significant decrease of HDL-cholesterol at 12 months. This unwanted decrease was absent in the group receiving a transdermal substitution 17β-estradiol (see Table 1). In the peroral group, there was a significant increase of HDL-cholesterol. Although there was – as expected – no HDL increase in the transdermal group, the HDL/LDL ratio passed into the favorable range because of the LDL decrease observed (values not shown in Table 1). In neither group was the ratio of HDL-2 to HDL-3 changed during the observation period. The pattern of the apolipoproteins A1, A2 and B is listed in the original publication[34].

Lipoprotein (a)

Neither in the control group nor in the two substituted groups receiving peroral or transdermal estrogens, did lipoprotein (a) show any significant changes[34]. However, there was a favorable trend towards a decrease of Lp (a) levels in both treatment groups. Therefore, this independent risk factor seems not to be primarily involved in the modification of the relative risk for cardiovascular diseases by estrogen substitution.

ADDITION OF A PROGESTAGEN: INFLUENCE ON SERUM LIPIDS

The addition of a progestagen[34,36] may influence the lipid changes induced by estrogens in the function of the type

Table 1 Comparison of a peroral (2 mg/day) with a transdermal (50 µg/day) administration of 17β-estradiol (continuous), combined with dydrogesterone (10 mg/day for 14 days each month). Determination of serum lipids was done before treatment (M-0) and at 6 ± 1 (M-6) and 12 ± 1 (M-12) months. Venous blood was drawn in the early morning after an overnight fasting period of 14 h on day 12–14 of the combined administration of estradiol and dydrogesterone. There was no statistical difference between the basal values of all lipids measured between the control group and the two substituted groups.

	n	Controls	n	Transdermal	n	Peroral
Triglycerides (mmol/l)						
M-0	35	1.09 ± 0.46	34	1.52 ± 0.99	34	1.34 ± 0.67
M-6	35	1.05 ± 0.40	33	1.35 ± 0.65	32	1.76 ± 0.95**††
M-12	34	1.07 ± 0.42	31	1.46 ± 1.27	31	1.68 ± 1.21*†
Total cholesterol (mmol/l)						
M-0	35	6.13 ± 1.18	34	6.68 ± 1.22	34	6.41 ± 1.23
M-6	35	6.03 ± 1.02	33	6.22 ± 0.80**	32	6.25 ± 1.16
M-12	34	6.24 ± 1.00†	31	6.42 ± 0.96*††	31	6.17 ± 0.98††
LDL-cholesterol (mmol/l)						
M-0	35	3.91 ± 0.98	34	4.49 ± 1.26	34	4.25 ± 1.37
M-6	35	3.85 ± 0.94	33	4.08 ± 0.74*††	32	3.74 ± 1.07***††
M-12	34	3.99 ± 0.91	31	4.13 ± 0.96**††	31	3.59 ± 0.86***†††
VLDL-cholesterol (mmol/l)						
M-0	35	0.40 ± 0.32	34	0.56 ± 0.53	n	0.52 ± 0.34
M-6	35	0.43 ± 0.34	33	0.59 ± 0.40	32	0.78 ± 0.51*†
M-12	34	0.49 ± 0.30	31	0.69 ± 0.70	31	0.82 ± 0.76*
HDL-cholesterol (mmol/l)						
M-0	35	1.81 ± 0.37	34	1.63 ± 0.50	34	0.29 ± 0.12
M-6	35	1.75 ± 0.37	33	1.56 ± 0.41	32	0.27 ± 0.10
M-12	34	1.76 ± 0.39*	31	1.60 ± 0.42	31	0.23 ± 0.07**†

Comparison within groups between basal, M-6 and M-12: *$p < 0.05$; **$p < 0.01$; ***$p < 0.001$
Comparison of the change between basal, M-6 and M-12 against controls: †$p < 0.05$; ††$p < 0.01$; †††$p < 0.001$

(particularly its androgenicity) and the dosage of the progestagen. In a simplified way, the derivatives of 17-hydroxyprogesterone (e.g. medroxyprogesterone acetate, medrogestone) are metabolically less potent than the derivatives of the 19-nortestosterone family (e.g. norethisterone acetate). The retrosteroids (e.g. dydrogesterone) are, judged by their effect on serum lipid levels, metabolically favorable as is by definition natural progesterone itself. The third-generation derivatives of the nortestosterone family (e.g. desogestrel, gestodene, norgestimate) can be considered to be favorable, too. In our study, dydrogesterone used in combination with 17β-estradiol did not neutralize the positive estrogenic effect (Table 1). The changes of serum lipids obtained with derivatives of 19-nortestosterone or with high doses of

medroxyprogesterone acetate were less favorable than those reported with dydrogesterone or natural progesterone, but they did not reverse the protective estrogen effect observed in the primate in vivo[37].

There was no change in lipoprotein (a), in controls or in the two treatment groups[34]. Because the serum levels of Lp (a) are primarily genetically determined and can remain constant for years in an individual, no conclusion can be drawn from the pattern of this independent risk factor during estrogen administration, in contrast to the changes of Lp (a) observed with tibolone[34]. However, the pattern of Lp (a) does not suggest an increase of the relative risk for cardiovascular diseases that might be induced by peroral or by transdermal estrogen substitution, with or without the addition of a progestagen.

HORMONE SUBSTITUTION: EFFECTS OF LONG-TERM ADMINISTRATION

Some data suggest that during prolonged postmenopausal hormonal substitution, the beneficial effect on serum lipids might be reduced[38]. Beginning after only 24 months of continuous hormone substitution, the positive as well as the negative changes induced by combined hormonal administration were reduced and less visible. However, the protective effect is lasting.

The PEPI Trial Writing Group[39] reports that peroral estrogens result in a significant HDL increase. Unopposed estrogens induce the highest increase with 5.6%. The second highest increase (4.1%) is observed with a combination of estrogens and micronized progesterone. In the PEPI Trial, the cumulative difference between the treatment and the placebo groups was highly significant ($p < 0.001$) although the placebo group had, too, a LDL decrease of 4.1%. If all treatment groups are pooled and compared to the placebo group, the mean HDL increase induced by estrogens is 5–6 mg/dl and the mean LDL-decrease 15 mg/dl. If 17β-estradiol is administered transdermally a similar pattern of lipid changes is observed[34], but in an attenuated form. The undesirable increase of triglycerides and VLDL induced by peroral estrogen administration can be avoided by transdermal estrogen administration. The decrease of LDL varies between 11% and 15% if 0.625 mg conjugated equine estrogens or 2 mg estradiol valerate are administered perorally, in transdermal administration it is less. The increase of HDL varies between 10–15% if 0.625 mg conjugated equine estrogens or 2 mg 17β-estradiol are administered perorally. Recent data show that women with total cholesterol levels superior to 240 mg/dl, but combined with HDL levels higher than 50 mg/dl do not possess an increased cardiovascular risk. In contrast, the risk is increased in women with total cholesterol levels of less than 200 mg/dl combined with HDL levels of less than 50 mg/dl. The cut-off-point of 50 mg/dl for HDL levels has in women with a HDL level of < 50 mg/dl the same predictive value as a HDL level of < 35 mg/dl in men[40,41]. The analysis of the observed LDL levels in three different groups (A, < 130; B, 130–159, and C, ≥ 160 mg/dl) show that in women, higher HDL levels are cardioprotective independent of the LDL and triglyceride levels measured. Estrogens modify the serum lipid pattern by decreasing the ratio LDL-cholesterol: HDL-cholesterol and the serum levels of lipoprotein(a). Both changes are considered to be cardioprotective.

SECONDARY CARDIOVASCULAR PREVENTION

Today, the benefit of primary cardiovascular prevention is clearly established. There is an absolute indication for estrogen–progestagen substitution in patients with an increased personal or familial cardiovascular risk (primary prevention). Although the evidence for secondary prevention is still quite poor, there are strong clinical, pathophysiological and experimental data in favor of secondary prevention[15–17,19]. In our opinion, the existing material is sufficient to recommend secondary prevention after myocardial infarction or in presence of a coronary disease. There are solid indications that women smoking cigarettes and patients suffering from arterial hypertension or having survived a first myocardial infarction may profit from hormonal substitution by conjugated estrogens or 17β-estradiol. This recommendation is in clear contradiction to our experience from oral contraception. However, in oral hormonal contraception, synthetic ethinylestradiol is used. Ethinyl-estradiol has a different metabolic pattern from that of natural estrogens and should not be used for hormonal substitution after menopause, in contrast to all natural estrogens. Unfortunately, this basic difference between synthetic and natural estrogens is not well enough known.

THE HERS TRIAL

The HERS trial is the first prospective randomized and controlled trial to study the effect of HRT on women with a preexisting coronary disease (secondary prevention). It has not been designed to study the effect of primary prevention. The study enrolled 2763 women with coronary heart disease. All women of the intervention group received the same fixed-combined HRT (conjugated equine estrogens plus MPA) in the same amount. The follow-up lasted on average 4.1 years. The primary endpoints have been coronarian death and non-fatal myocardial infarction. The HERS study does not include a study group using estrogens alone. Therefore, the results of the HERS study have to be analyzed in function of the progestagen used in combination with conjugated estrogens. The outcome of the HERS study[42] might have been mainly determined by the choice of the progestagen MPA. If this hypothesis is true it has to be confirmed by other trials. The results of the HERS trial consist of a nonsignificant increase in coronary death (hazard ratio 1.24 (0.8–1.75)), a non-significant decrease in non-fatal myocardial infarction (0.91 (0.71–1.17) and a significant increase in thomboembolic events (2.89 (1.50–5.58). However, the trial is characterized by several weak points; the drop-out rate was greater than expected, particularly in the substituted group. In the control group, the rate of fatal events was lower (3.3% versus 5%), and, in HRT users, the occurrence of thromboembolic events higher than expected from other studies in postmenopausal women. But, most intriguing, the analysis of the drop-outs revealed that 110 controls (8% of all controls) compared to only 36 drop-outs (3% of all HRT users) admitted to receiving HRT from another source, independently from the trial. A subanalysis of the group of women taking only the medication allocated by randomization resulted in a non-significant beneficial effect of HRT (0.87 (0.67–1.11)). Furthermore, the risk of cardiovascular death decreased to 0.67 (hazard ratio) in years 4 and 5 of the study, pointing to a clear long-term benefit of HRT in women suffering from coronary disease, an aspect neglected in the discussion of the first analysis of this important trial.

CONCLUSION

For years, the cardioprotective effect of estrogens has been explained by their favorable influence on the lipid profile[41,43,44]. However, the results of the Lipid Research Clinics Program and other newer data suggest that the changes of the lipid profile participate in about 20–30% of the reduction of the cardiovascular risk[40,45], and it has been accepted that the direct estrogenic effect at the arterial wall is responsible for 70–80% of the cardioprotection by ERT. The administration of estrogens leads to an arterial dilation through a direct effect on the vascular wall. This effect is maintained in atherosclerotic coronary arteries.

Several epidemiological studies have shown that hormonal substitution reduces the cardiovascular risk after menopause significantly, by about 50%. Although the direct estrogen effect at the arterial endothelium contributes to a great extent to the total estrogen benefit, the favorable serum lipid changes play an important role. Our own observation as well as newer data from the literature show that in the transdermal route of estrogen administration the decrease of plasma LDL levels is smaller than in the peroral route. However, in the transdermal route of administration, too, LDL-cholesterol decreases and HDL increases significantly. The slight decrease of Lp (a) in the peroral and the transdermal treatment groups suggests a positive effect of estrogen substitution on the cardiovascular risk. Our data lead to the conclusion that the combined administration of 17β-estradiol and dydrogesterone induce a favorable change in the plasma lipid pattern.

From the literature, it can be postulated that the peroral administration of small amounts of the derivatives of 17-hydroxyprogesterone do not neutralize the beneficial effects of natural estrogens. However, to date, all important studies have been done in healthy women presenting a normal lipid profile. The response to hormonal substitution in women with pathological lipid levels is not well documented. Animal data show that norethisterone acetate does not reverse the positive effect of 17β-estradiol observed directly at the arterial endothelium.

In conclusion, there are no data in healthy women which indicate that a certain hormonal combination or a specific route of administration is clearly superior or clearly inferior to other substances or other routes of administration. However, a more specific analysis of the effects of well-defined estrogen–progestagen combinations is needed for primary and for secondary prevention of cardiovascular diseases.

Although epidemiological observational studies may present some weaknesses, there is no reason to change our opinions on the indication of HRT prescribed for primary prevention in women at high risk for cardiovascular disease. The HERS trial[42] cannot be used to decide on primary prevention of coronary disease because the trial has been designed for secondary prevention. However, the situation might be more complex if estrogens are used for secondary cardiovascular prevention as has been done in the HERS trial[42]. The, in part, unexpected and contradictory results of this study might be linked to some weaknesses of the study design, such as the short follow-up period, the unexpected and uncontrolled estrogen use in the drop-outs, and to the specific progestagen used in the treatment regimen rather than to the administration of the estrogen only. But it also has to be considered that women suffering from coronary heart disease might be a negative selection, more prone to some complications, such as thromboembolic events, than the general population.

References

1. Johansson BW, Kaü L, Kullander S, et al. On some late effects of bilateral oophorectomy in the age range 15–30 years. Acta Obstet Gynecol Scand 1975; 54:449–61
2. Wuest J, Dry T, Edwards J. The degree of coronary atherosclerosis in bilaterally oophorectomized women. Circulation 1953;7: 801–9
3. Kannel WV, Hjortland M, McNamara PM, et al. Menopause and risk of cardiovascular disease: the Framingham study. Ann Intern Med 1976;85: 447–552
4. Robinson RW, Higano N, Cohen WO. Increased incidence of coronary heart disease in women castrated prior to menopause. Arch Int Med 1959;104:980
5. Bush TL, Fried LP, Barrett-Connor E. Cholesterol, lipoproteins, and coronary heart disease in women. Clin Chem 1988;34:B60
6. Stampfer MJ, Colditz GA, Willett WC. Menopause and heart disease. In Flint M, Kronenberg F, Utian W, eds. Multidisciplinary Perspectives on Menopause. Ann NY Arch Sci 1990;592
7. Colditz GA, Willet WC, Stampfer MJ, et al. Menopause and the risk of coronary heart disease in women. N Engl J Med 1987;316:1105
8. Sarrel PM. Ovarian hormones and the circulation. Maturitas 1990;12:287
9. Sullivan JM, Vander-Zwaag R, Lemp GF, et al. Postmenopausal estrogen use and coronary atherosclerosis. Ann Intern Med 1988;108:358
10. Rosano GMC, Crea F. Chest pain and myocardial ischemia in syndrome X: new pathogenetic hypotheses. Coron Arterial Dis 1992;3:599
11. Rosano GMC, Lindsay DC, Kaski JC, et al. Syndrome X in women: the importance of the ovarian hormones (Abstract). J Am Coll Cardiol 1992;19:255
12. Sarrel PM, Lindsay D, Rosano GMC, et al. Angina and normal coronary arteries: gynecologic findings. Am J Obstet Gynecol 1992;167:467–72
13. Osler W. Lectures on Angina Pectoris and Allied States. New York: Appleton, 1901
14. LaCroix AZ, Haynes SG, Savage DD, et al. Rose questionnaire angina among United States black, white and Mexican-American women, and men. Am J Epidemiol 1989;129:669
15. Rosano GMC, Sarrel PM, Poole-Wilson PA, et al. Beneficial effect of oestrogen on exercise-induced myocardial ischaemia in women with coronary artery disease. Lancet 1993;342:133–6
16. Rosano GMC, Sarrel PM, Poole-Wilson PA, et al. Effects of acute administration of estradiol-17-beta on exercise-induced myocardial ischemia in female patients with coronary artery disease. Lancet 1993;342:133

17. Williams JK, Adams MR, Klopfenstein S. Estrogen modulates responses of atherosclerotic coronary arteries. *Circulation* 1990;81:1680

18. Pines A, Fisman EZ, Levo Y, *et al.* The effects of hormone replacement therapy in normal postmenopausal women: measurements of Doppler derived parameters of aortic flow. *Am J Obstet Gynecol* 1991;164:806

19. Collins P, Rosano GMC, Jiang C, *et al.* Cardiovascular protection by estrogen – a calcium antagonist effect? *Lancet* 1993;341:1264

20. Polderman KH, Stehouwer CDA, van Kamp GJ, *et al.* Influence of sex hormones on plasma endothelin levels. *Ann Intern Med* 1993;118:429

21. Chang WC, Nakao J, Orimo H, *et al.* Stimulation of prostacyclin biosynthesis activity by estradiol in rat aortic smooth muscle cells in culture. *Biochim Biophys Acta* 1980;619:107

22. Fogelberg M, Vesterquist O, Diczfalusey U, *et al.* Experimental atherosclerosis effects of oestrogen and atherosclerosis on thromboxane and prostacyclin formation. *Eur J Clin Invest* 1990; 20:105

23. Jiang C, Sarrel PM, Lindsay DC, *et al.* Endothelium independent relaxation of rabbit coronary artery by 17-beta-estradiol in vitro. *Br J Pharmacol* 1991;104:1033

24. Jiang C, Sarrel PM, Poole-Wilson PA, *et al.* Acute effects of 17β-estradiol on rabbit coronary artery contractile response to endothelin. *Am J Physiol* 1992;263 (*Heart Circ Physiol* 32):H271

25. Herrington DM, Braden GA, Downes TR, *et al.* Estrogen modulates coronary vasomotor responses in postmenopausal women with early atherosclerosis. *Circulation* 1992;1–619 (Abstract 2461)

26. Notelovitz M, Gudat JC, Ware MW, *et al.* Lipids and lipoproteins in women after oophorectomy and the response to estrogen therapy. *Br J Obstet Gynaecol* 1983;90:171

27. Campagnoli C, Tousijn P, Belforte P, *et al.* Effect of conjugated equine estrogens and estriol on blood clotting, plasma lipids and endometrial proliferation in postmenopausal women. *Maturitas* 1981;3:135

28. Fahraeus L, Larsson-Cohn U, Wallentin L. Lipoproteins during oral and cutaneous administration of estradiol-17-beta to menopausal women. *Acta Endocrinol (Copenh)* 1982;101:597

29. Bush TL, Millter VT. Effects of pharmacologic agents used during menopause: impact on lipids and lipoproteins. In Mishell DR, ed. *Menopause: Physiology and Pharmacology.* Chicago: Year Book Medical Publishers, 1989:187

30. Lobo RA. Effects of hormone replacement on lipids and lipoproteins in postmenopausal women. *J Clin Endocrinol Metab* 1991;73:925

31. Elkik F, Gompel A, Mercier-Bodard C, *et al.* Effects of percutaneous estradiol and conjugated estrogens on the level of plasma proteins and triglycerides in postmenopausal women. *Am J Obstet Gynecol* 1982;143:888

32. Enk L, Crona N, Samsioe G, *et al.* Dose and duration effects of estradiol valerate on serum and lipoprotein lipids. *Horm Metab Res* 1986; 18:551

33. Chetkowski RJ, Meldrum DR, Steingold KA, *et al.* Biologic effects of transdermal estradiol. *N Engl Med* 1986;314:1615

34. Hänggi W, Lippuner K, Riesen W, *et al.* Long-term influence of different hormone replacement regimens on serum lipids and lipoprotein (a): a randomised study. *Br J Obstet Gynaecol* 1997;104:708–17

35. Cauly JA, LePorte RE, Kuller LH, *et al.* Menopausal estrogen use, high density lipoprotein cholesterol subfractions and liver function. *Atherosclerosis* 1983;49:31

36. Wolfe, BM, Huff MW. Effects of combined estrogen and progestin administration on plasma lipoprotein metabolism in postmenopausal women. *J Clin Invest* 1989;83:40

37. Adams MR, Williams JK, Clarkson TB, et al. Effects of estrogens and progestogens on coronary atherosclerosis and osteoporosis of monkeys. *Baillière's Clin Obstet Gynaecol* 1991;5:915

38. Jensen J, Riis BJ, Ström V, *et al.* Long-term and withdrawal effects of two different estrogen-progestogen combinations on lipid and lipoprotein profiles in postmenopausal women. *Maturitas* 1989;11:117

39. PEPI Trial Writing Group. Effects of estrogen or estrogen/progestin regimes on heart disease risk factors in postmenopausal women: the postmenopausal Estrogen/Progestin Interventions (PEPI) Trial. *J Am Med Assoc* 1995;273: 199–208

40. Bush TL, Barrett-Conner E, Cowan LD, *et al.* Cardiovascular mortality and noncontraceptive use of oestrogen in women: results from the Lipid Research Clinics Program Follow-up Study. *Circulation* 1987;75:1102–9

41. Bass KM, Newschaffer CJ, Klag MJ, *et al.* Plasma lipoprotein levels as predictors of cardiovascular death in women. *Arch Intern Med* 1993;153:2209–16

42. Hulley St, Grady D, Bush T, *et al.*, for the Heart and Estrogen/progestin Replacement Study (HERS) Research Group. Randomized trial of estrogen plus progestin for secondary prevention of coronary heart disease in postmenopausal women. *J Am Med Assoc* 1998;280:605–13

43. Mautner SL, Lin F, Mautner GC, *et al.* Comparison in women versus men of composition of atherosclerotic plaques in native coronary arteries and in saphenous veins used as aortocoronary conduits. *J Am Coll Cardiol* 1993;71:1312–8

44. Clarkson TB, Adams MR, Williams JK, *et al.* Effects of sex steroids on the monkey cardiovascular system: relation to changes in serum lipids and lipoproteins. In Christiansen C, Overgaard K, eds. *Osteoporosis* 1990:1798–805

45. Stampfer MJ, Colditz GA. Estrogen replacement therapy and coronary heart disease: a quantitative assessment of the epidemiologic evidence. *Prev Med* 1991;20:47-63

The impact of progestin on the cardiovascular benefits of estrogen 12

F. Grodstein and M.J. Stampfer

BACKGROUND

Cardiovascular diseases remain the leading cause of death in women in industrialized countries. Estrogen use by postmenopausal women has been associated with a decrease in rates of coronary heart disease (CHD) in over 30 epidemiologic studies[1]; the summary relative risk from all of these studies combined indicates that current hormone users may have a 50% lower risk of heart disease than never users. However, in most studies, the vast majority of women used conjugated estrogen alone; more recently, progestins have been prescribed along with estrogen to women with an intact uterus to reduce or eliminate the excess risk of endometrial cancer due to unopposed estrogen. In this review, based on a previous manuscript we have published[2], we evaluate the data regarding the impact of added progestin on cardiovascular disease risk, including the biological and epidemiological evidence.

BIOLOGICAL MECHANISMS

Substantial biological data support a role for estrogen in preventing CHD. The best established mechanism is estrogen's impact on the lipid profile[3]. In experimental studies among postmenopausal women, estrogen reduced low-density lipoprotein (LDL) and raised high-density lipoprotein (HDL). However, progestins tend to raise LDL and lower HDL, and may thus detract from the beneficial effect of estrogens on the lipid profile.

Miller and colleagues[4] found that the estrogen-induced increase in HDL was attenuated by 14–17% with progestin use, but there was little change on the reduction of LDL. These effects differ by type of progestin. In the Postmenopausal Estrogen and Progestin Intervention Trial[5], five groups of 175 women each were randomized for 3 years to placebo, oral estrogen alone, oral estrogen plus cyclic or continuous medroxyprogesterone acetate (MPA), or oral estrogen with cyclic micronized progesterone. Significant increases in HDL and decreases in LDL were found for all treatment groups compared to placebo. Comparable decreases in LDL were observed for all hormone regimens (by 0.37–0.46 mmol/l), although for HDL, the elevation among users of estrogen with MPA (by 0.03–0.04 mmol/l) was less than that for users of estrogen alone (increase of 0.14 mmol/l) or estrogen with micronized progestin (0.11 mmol/l).

In animal studies examining the effect of added progestin on cholesterol accumulation in the arteries, the results also vary by type of hormone, although relatively few investigations have been conducted. Rabbits given norethisterone acetate or levonorgestrel with estradiol, or estradiol alone, all had similarly reduced aortic accumulation of cholesterol (by one-third) compared to a placebo group[6]. Monkeys administered either estrogen with progesterone or estrogen alone also had similarly decreased LDL accumulation in the coronary arteries (by 70%)[7] and less atherosclerosis (50% reduction)[8] than those on placebo. In monkeys given MPA with conjugated equine estrogen, however, the extent of atherosclerosis was similar to those given placebo and greater than in monkeys taking estrogen alone[9].

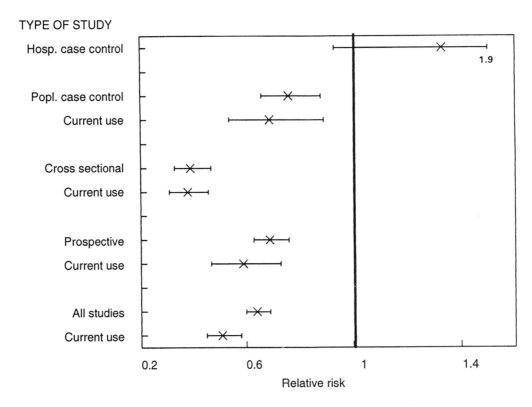

Figure 1   Heart disease and postmenopausal hormones: meta-analysis of ever and current use

Estrogen therapy also improves blood flow, but limited studies suggest that this benefit may be diminished with the addition of progestin. In ovariectomized ewes, a 20–30% decrease in uterine blood flow was observed when progesterone was added to estradiol; subsequent withdrawal of progesterone was followed by a sharp increase in blood flow[10]. Sullivan and co-workers[11] reported that 10 mg of MPA given for 10 days with oral conjugated estrogen led to a significant rise in forearm vascular resistance among six postmenopausal women. In 12 women given micronized 17-β estradiol with 1 mg norethisterone acetate daily, the pulsatility index was significantly reduced after 4 months of treatment[12].

EPIDEMIOLOGICAL EVIDENCE

Nearly all epidemiological studies have observed an inverse relationship between estrogen use and heart disease. In a meta-analysis of all of the epidemiological studies assessing ever versus never use, with relative risks ranging from 0.17 to 4.2, we calculated a summary relative risk of 0.65 (95% CI 0.60–0.70)[1] (Figure 1). However, evidence from many of these studies indicates that current estrogen users enjoy greater protection against heart disease than past users; therefore, combining investigations of current, past and ever use in a summary estimate such as this may be misleading. We re-calculated summary estimates based on analyses of current use, where such data were provided, and as expected these estimates were more marked than those produced by combining studies of any estrogen use (Figure 1). The pooled relative risk for current estrogen use was 0.49 (95% CI 0.43–0.56).

Progestin use was uncommon during the period that most of the epidemiologic studies were conducted and data on its effect on CHD risk are relatively sparse, although available data indicate that adding progestin does not eliminate the cardiovascular benefits of hormone therapy (Table 1). In a case–control study with 502 cases of myocardial infarction (MI) and 1193 controls, Psaty and colleagues[13] reported relative risks of 0.68 (95% CI 0.38–1.22) for current users of estrogen with progestin (MPA) and 0.69 (95% CI 0.47–1.02) for users of estrogen alone. Using the entire population of Uppsala, Sweden, Falkeborn and associates[14] also found that MI was reduced by 47% (RR = 0.53, 95% CI 0.30–0.87) in women taking estrogen with a progestin (levonorgestrel, MPA and norethisterone acetate) and 31% (0.54–0.86) in those taking estrogen alone. In a recent report from the Nurses' Health Study[15], with 60 000 subjects and 770 cases of MI, the risks were diminished for women using estrogen with progestin (primarily MPA, RR = 0.39, 95% CI 0.19–0.78) or estrogen alone (RR = 0.60, 95% CI 0.43–0.83).

Nonetheless, with the exception of one small clinical trial in which one of 84 women given estrogen with progestin and three untreated women had an MI over 10 years of follow-up (RR = 0.3)[16], all of the epidemiologic evidence accumulated to date is from observational studies. In the observational studies, it is the participants and their physicians who decide whether to use hormone therapy. Often the health status of the patient has an important influence on this decision. In addition, women who use estrogen see a physician more regularly than those who do not, and this increased medical care may decrease their risk of CHD. Furthermore, women who choose to use hormones may also choose to lead generally healthier lifestyles than those who do not take such medication. Therefore, some have argued that hormone use is merely a marker, rather than a cause, of good health. Most of the studies have provided some information bearing on this critical point[17].

In the Nurses' Health Study[15], we assessed whether increased medical care among hormone users could be responsible for the benefit observed. Only women who reported a recent physician visit (50% of the cohort) were included in the analysis, and the results were similar to those found in all subjects; the relative risk for major coronary heart disease was 0.52 (95% CI 0.37–0.74) for current use.

Several studies have compared the CHD risk factor profile of estrogen users and non-users. In general population studies, estrogen

Table 1 Epidemiological studies of postmenopausal use of estrogen and progestin

Study	Design	n	Results
Psaty et al.[13] Group Health Cooperative of Puget Sound	case–control	502 MI cases 1193 controls	RR = 0.69 (95% CI 0.47–1.02) current estrogen alone RR = 0.68 (95% CI 0.38–1.22) current combined therapy
Falkeborn et al.[14] Uppsala, Sweden	prospective	227 MI cases 23 174 women	RR = 0.74 (95% CI 0.61–0.88) ever estrogen alone RR = 0.50 (95% CI 0.28–0.80) ever combined therapy
Grodstein et al.[15] Nurses' Health Study	prospective	770 MI cases 59 337 women	RR = 0.60 (95% CI 0.43–0.83) current estrogen alone RR = 0.39 (95% CI 0.19–0.78) current combined therapy
Nachtigall et al.[16]	clinical trial	4 MI cases 168 women	RR = 0.33 (95% CI 0.04–2.82) current combined therapy

MI, myocardial infarction; RR, relative risk

users appear to have a more favorable cardiac risk profile than non-users, even apart from hormone use. However, in many of the large studies, the subjects tend to be quite homogeneous, chosen because of their common profession or community. In the Nurses' Health Study[15], the Lipid Research Clinics Follow-up Study[18] and the Leisure World Study[19], the distribution of coronary risk factors was similar among current and never users of hormones, although the users tended to be somewhat leaner and more physically active. In these investigations, multivariate control for numerous risk factors had little impact on the relative risk estimates for hormones and heart disease, implying a nearly equivalent risk status for users and non-users. In summary, to explain the benefit as a result of confounding, one would have to presume unknown risk factors which are extremely strong predictors of CHD and very closely associated with hormone use.

CONCLUSIONS

The decision to use hormone therapy is perhaps the most complex medical decision that any normal healthy menopausal woman typically faces. Long-term hormone therapy may increase the risk of breast cancer[20]. However, the benefits of reducing menopausal symptoms and decreasing bone loss are well-established, and the evidence that estrogen protects against heart disease is quite strong. While the biological data regarding progestin's effects on the cardiovascular system are not completely clear, at least some of the lipid benefits are maintained, and, in the few epidemiological studies to date, women taking estrogen with progestin appear to have a similar decrease in risk to those taking estrogen alone.

References

1. Grodstein F, Stampfer MJ. The epidemiology of coronary heart disease and estrogen replacement in postmenopausal women. *Prog Cardiol Dis* 1995;3:199–210
2. Grodstein F, Stampfer MJ. The impact of progestin on estrogen's cardiovascular benefits. *Menopause Manage* 1997;6:10–16
3. Bush TL, Miller VT. Effects of pharmacologic agents used during menopause. Impact on lipids and lipoproteins. In Mishell D, ed. *Menopause: Physiology and Pharmacology*. Chicago: Year Book Medical Publishers, 1986:187–208
4. Miller VT, Muesing RA, LaRosa JC, *et al.* Effects of conjugated equine estrogen with and without three different progestogens on lipoproteins, high-density lipoprotein subfractions, and apolipoprotein A-1. *Obstet Gynecol* 1991;77:235
5. Postmenopausal Estrogen/Progestin Interventions Trial Writing Group. Effects of estrogen/progestin regimens on heart disease risk factors in postmenopausal women. *J Am Med Assoc* 1995;273:199–208
6. Haarbo J, Leth-Espensen P, Stender S, *et al.* Estrogen monotherapy and combined estrogen-progestogen replacement therapy attenuate aortic accumulation of cholesterol in ovariectomized cholesterol-fed rabbits. *J Clin Invest* 1991;87:1274–9
7. Wagner JD, Clarkson TB, St Clair RW, *et al.* Estrogen and progesterone replacement therapy reduces low density lipoprotein accumulation in the coronary arteries of surgically postmenopausal cyno-molgus monkeys. *J Clin Invest* 1991;88:1995–2002
8. Adams MR, Kaplan JR, Manuck SB, *et al.* Inhibition of coronary artery atherosclerosis by 17-beta estradiol in ovariectomized monkeys. Lack of an effect of added progesterone. *Arteriosclerosis* 1990;10:1051–7
9. Adams MR, Golden DL. Atheroprotective effects of estrogen replacement therapy are antagonized by medroxyprogesterone acetate in monkeys [Abstract]. *Circulation* 1995;92(Suppl. 1):627
10. Sarrel PM. Blood flow. In Lobo R, ed. *Treatment of the Postmenopausal Woman*. New York: Raven Press, 1994:251–62
11. Sullivan JM, Shala BA, Miller LA, *et al.* Progestin enhances vasoconstrictor responses in postmenopausal women receiving estrogen replacement therapy. *Menopause* 1995;2:193–9

12. Gangar KF, McCullogh W, Penny J, *et al.* Continuous combined hormone replacement therapy and cardiovascular protection. *Eur Menopause J* 1996;3:147–50

13. Psaty BM, Heckbert SR, Atkins D, *et al.* The risk of myocardial infarction associated with the combined use of estrogens and progestins in postmenopausal women. *Arch Intern Med* 1994;154:1333–9

14. Falkeborn M, Persson I, Adami HO, *et al.* The risk of acute myocardial infarction after oestrogen and oestrogen–progestogen replacement. *Br J Obstet Gynaecol* 1992;99:821–8

15. Grodstein F, Stampfer MJ, Manson JE, *et al.* Postmenopausal estrogen and progestin use and the risk of cardiovascular disease. *N Engl J Med* 1996;335:453–61

16. Nachtigall LE, Nachtigall RH, Nachtigall RD, *et al.* Estrogen replacement therapy II: a prospective study in the relationship to carcinoma and cardiovascular metabolic problems. *Obstet Gynecol* 1979;54:74–9

17. Grodstein F. Can selection bias explain the cardiovascular benefits of estrogen replacement therapy? [Editorial] *Am J Epidemiol* 1996;143:979–82

18. Bush TL, Barrett-Connor E, Cowan LD, *et al.* Cardiovascular mortality and noncontraceptive use of estrogen in women: results from the Lipid Research Clinics Program Follow-up Study. *Circulation* 1987;75:1102–9

19. Henderson BE, Paganini-Hill A, Ross RK. Decreased mortality in users of estrogen replacement therapy. *Arch Intern Med* 1991;151:75–8

20. Colditz GA, Hankinson SE, Hunter DJ, *et al.* The use of estrogens and progestins and the risk of breast cancer in postmenopausal women. *N Engl J Med* 1995;332:1589–93

Hormone replacement therapy and insulin resistance

13

S.O. Skouby

The epidemiological evidence for the association between deterioration of glucose tolerance and cardiovascular disease (CVD) has been documented in several investigations. It is also a well-known fact that glucose tolerance decreases with age and concomitantly with the appearance of other elements from the metabolic syndrome of insulin resistance. These facts, combined with the experience from reproductive biology that endogenous and exogenous sex steroids can modulate glucose metabolism, make it of obvious interest to investigate whether the preventive effect of hormonal replacement therapy (HRT) on CVD can be explained, at least partly, through its effect on glucose tolerance.

Both beta-cell dysfunction and insulin resistance are responsible for the decrease in glucose intolerance with increasing age, whereas body fat, changes in insulin clearance or insulin-dependent glucose disappearance seem to be of only minor importance. Hyperglycemia with accompanying hyperinsulinemia damages or alters the endothelial barrier, allowing insulin to interact with underlying smooth muscle cells. As a result, proliferation and migration of the cells occurs and they accumulate lipid due to increased lipogenesis.

Most of our knowledge about the effect of different sex steroid combinations on glucose metabolism has been obtained from the oral contraceptive area. With these preparations hyperinsulinemia is often observed following an oral glucose tolerance test (OGTT) indicating increased insulin resistance. No influence on the OGTT from unopposed estrogen treatment with natural estrogens has, however, been demonstrated, and, more recently, it has been demonstrated that fasting insulin values, a reliable marker for insulin sensitivity, are lower among users of estrogen compared to untreated postmenopausal women. Thus, natural estrogens may reduce insulin resistance and thereby prevent formation of atherosclerotic plaques. The impact of HRT is, however, modulated according to the route of hormone administration and the progestin addition. Long-term HRT studies on insulin sensitivity with proper adjustments for these factors as well as for confounding factors such as obesity, blood pressure, lipoprotein levels, exercise and diet are therefore needed before a proper conclusion can be drawn on the inter-relationship between HRT, insulin and CVD.

Body composition and cyclical changes in serum lipids and lipoproteins during combined hormone replacement therapy

14

J. Haarbo

INTRODUCTION

Serum lipids and lipoproteins are important cardiovascular risk factors in women[1]. It is well known that postmenopausal estrogen monotherapy induces a beneficial increase in high-density lipoprotein cholesterol (HDL-C) and a decrease in the atherogenic lipoprotein low-density lipoprotein cholesterol (LDL-C)[2]. Progestogens generally have an adverse lowering effect on HDL-C. Sequential addition of a progestogen to estrogen replacement therapy may therefore induce cyclical changes in serum lipids and lipoproteins during the tablet cycle.

Increased body weight is also associated with cardiovascular risk. Many postmenopausal women complain about weight gain in the postmenopausal years and blame hormone replacement therapy (HRT) for that undesired change. But does HRT increase body weight? And what happens to body fat distribution, which seems to be more closely related to cardiovascular disease than to body fat *per se*.

CYCLICAL CHANGES IN SERUM LIPIDS AND LIPOPROTEINS DURING HRT

We have data from a dose–response study (1,2 or 4 mg estradiol sequentially combined with 1 mg norethisterone acetate), which clearly demonstrate cyclical changes in HDL-C with a dose-dependent increase during the estrogen-only period and a fall during the combined period[3]. The HDL-C concentration

is therefore dependent on the time of blood sampling. To obtain the best estimate of the impact of a hormone combination on HDL-C, one should ideally integrate the area under the curve based on frequent HDL-C measurements. We measured serum lipids and lipoproteins initially and 16 times during two consecutive cycles (56 days) in the above-mentioned study. The 'true' area under the curve based on all 16 measurements could accurately be estimated by two determinations per cycle taken at the end of the estrogen and estrogen/progestogen periods, respectively[4]. It is therefore possible to adjust for cyclical changes in serum lipids and lipoproteins if two determinations taken at such time points are available. Moreover, this procedure may improve comparisons between different sequentially combined regimens, especially if correction for changes in a parallel placebo group is included.

We designed a study in which 148 healthy early postmenopausal women were randomized to two groups 6 months apart[4]. The women in the first group were randomly assigned to receive 2 mg estradiol valerate either continuously, combined with 1 mg cyproterone acetate, or sequentially, with 75 μg levonorgestrel, or placebo. The women in the second group were randomized to receive estradiol sequentially, combined with either 150 μg desogestrel, or 10 mg medroxyprogesterone acetate, or placebo.

Serum lipids and lipoproteins were measured initially and during the following

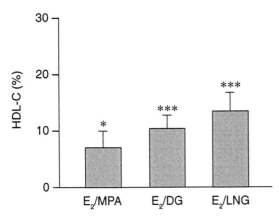

Figure 1 The significant cyclical variations in high-density lipoprotein-cholesterol (HDL-C) after correction for placebo, shown for the initial 84 days of the study for the three combined hormone regimens. E_2, estradiol; MPA, medroxyprogesterone acetate; DG, desogestrel; LNG, levonorgestrel. *$p < 0.05$; ***$p < 0.001$

three cycles at the end of the estrogen-only and combined estrogen/progestogen period. These sampling points were the same as those found to be optimal in the above mentioned initial 'cyclical' study. Figure 1 shows the cyclical variations (estrogen-related value minus estrogen/progestogen-related value) in the three sequential groups after correction for changes in the placebo group. Similar changes were seen in apolipoprotein A_1 and, as expected, there were no significant changes in the continuous combined group. At the end of the 2-year study period cyclical variations were similar to those found during the initial 84 days[5].

To obtain the true response to treatment it is important to correct not only for cyclical changes but also for the changes that occur in the corresponding placebo group. This may eliminate seasonal variations in serum lipids and lipoproteins as well as 'trial-induced' changes in diet and physical activity. After placebo correction, all four regimens were found to induce a beneficial reduction in LDL-C of about 6–14% with no significant differences between groups. Similar reductions were seen in total cholesterol and apolipoprotein B, the principal apolipoprotein of the LDL particle. There were no

significant overall changes in HDL-C or apolipoprotein A_1. These findings indicate that:

(1) Sequential HRT may induce significant cyclical changes in serum lipids and lipoproteins, especially HDL-C and apolipoprotein A_1, as long as therapy is given;

(2) Comparison of different sequential regimens should ideally include correction for cyclical changes;

(3) Following of serum lipids and lipoproteins in an individual woman on sequential HRT should be based on samples taken during the same time of the tablet phase.

BODY COMPOSITION

It is well known that body weight increases with age and this rise seems to be most pronounced in the third and fourth decade[6]. Whether the weight increase is higher in postmenopausal women as compared to age-matched premenopausal controls is controversial[6–8]. We have performed several randomized, double-blind and placebo-controlled studies where we have looked at the impact of HRT on body weight. In these studies, HRT-treated early postmenopausal women tended to gain less body weight than postmenopausal women on placebo[8]. This underlines the fact that HRT is not the reason for the postmenopausal weight increase, which is due to changes in energy expenditure[9].

Body fat distribution seems to be more closely related to cardiovascular risk than body weight *per se*. We therefore evaluated the impact of combined HRT on abdominal fat percentage[10]. This study included 75 early postmenopausal women who were randomized to either combined HRT or placebo for 2 years. There was a tendency towards a lower increase in total body fat in the hormone group as compared to the women in the placebo group. The hormone group

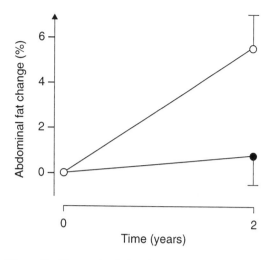

Figure 2 Change in abdominal fat percentage in the placebo group (open circles) and the combined hormone (estrogen/progestogen) group (filled circles)

also seemed to preserve lean tissue mass better than the placebo group; however, these differences were not statistically significant. In contrast, the significant increase in abdominal fat percentage seen in the placebo group was prevented in the combined hormone group (Figure 2). These findings indicate that:

(1) Body weight increases in the perimenopausal years;

(2) HRT prevents the postmenopausal increase in abdominal fat;

(3) HRT seems to preserve the premenopausal lean to fat ratio.

References

1. Castelli WP, Garrison RJ, Wilson PWF, *et al.* Incidence of coronary heart disease and lipoprotein cholesterol levels. The Framingham Study. *J Am Med Assoc* 1986;256:2835–8

2. Nabulsi AA, Folsom AR, White A, *et al.* Association of hormone-replacement therapy with various cardiovascular risk factors in post menopausal women. *N Engl J Med* 1993;328:1069–75

3. Jensen J, Nilas L, Christiansen C. Cyclic changes in serum cholesterol and lipoproteins following different doses of combined postmenopausal hormone replacement therapy. *Br J Obstet Gynaecol* 1986;93:613–8

4. Haarbo J, Hassager C, Jensen SB, *et al.* Serum lipids, lipoproteins, and apolipoproteins during postmenopausal replacement therapy combined with either 19-nortestosterone derivatives or 17-hydroxy-progesterone derivatives. *Am J Med* 1991;90:584–9

5. Haarbo J, Christiansen C. Treatment-induced cyclic variations in serum lipids, lipoproteins, and apolipoproteins after 2 years of combined hormone replacement therapy: exaggerated cyclic variations in smokers. *Obstet Gynecol* 1992;80:639–44

6. Heymsfield SB, Gallagher D, Poehlman ET, *et al.* Menopausal changes in body composition and energy expenditure. *Exp Geront* 1994;29:377–89

7. Wang Q, Hassager C, Ravn P, *et al.* Total and regional body-composition changes in early postmenopausal women: age-related or menopause-related? *Am J Clin Nutr* 1994;60:843–8

8. Hassager C. Soft tissue body composition during prevention and treatment of postmenopausal osteoporosis assessed by photon absorptiometry (Thesis). *Dan Med Bull* 1991;38:380–9

9. Poehlman ET, Toth MJ, Gardner AW. Changes in energy balance and body composition at menopause: a controlled longitudinal study. *Ann Intern Med* 1995;123:673–5

10. Haarbo J, Marslew U, Gotfredsen A, *et al.* Postmenopausal hormone replacement therapy prevents central distribution of body fat after menopause. *Metabolism* 1991;40:1323–6

HRT and atherosclerosis: studies in cholesterol-fed rabbits

15

J. Haarbo

INTRODUCTION

Since Anitschkow at the beginning of this century began to use rabbits for studies of experimental atherosclerosis, this model has been used in numerous investigations of various aspects of atherosclerosis. The fat- or cholesterol-fed rabbit has many advantages over other species, as it is easily handled, comparatively inexpensive, breeds well and reliably develops lipid rich fatty streaks on exposure to cholesterol. One important drawback in using the cholesterol-fed rabbit is that the lipid and lipoprotein profiles in plasma do not resemble those of humans. On the other hand, the lesions of fat-fed rabbits and Watanabe heritable hyperlipidemic rabbits (WHHL) have many similarities such as a comparable distribution of various cells within lesions and a similar capacity to incorporate thymidine into proliferating cells[1]. As the disease in WHHL rabbits closely mimics the accelerated disease seen in familial hypercholesterolemia, it is generally accepted that the cholesterol-fed rabbit is a useful model for the study of atherosclerosis[2].

STUDIES OF FEMALE SEX HORMONES IN CHOLESTEROL-FED RABBITS

Early studies[3–5] indicated an anti-atherogenic effect of estrogens and a lowering influence on plasma lipids. Kushwaha and Hazzard[6] showed that intramuscularly injected estradiol was able to attenuate diet-induced atherosclerosis in comparison to the condition of control rabbits. Their study also suggested that

this beneficial effect in part was mediated through the lowering of very low-density lipoprotein (VLDL)- and intermediate-density lipoprotein (IDL)-cholesterol. A controlled study in 32 white New Zealand rabbits[7] demonstrated that ovariectomized cholesterol-fed rabbits had a significantly greater degree of atherosclerosis than a group with intact ovaries. Two other groups of rabbits were ovariectomized, cholesterol-fed and injected intramuscularly with either estradiol or progesterone weekly. The estradiol-treated rabbits had a degree of atherosclerosis that was similar to that of rabbits with intact ovaries, whereas progesterone-treated rabbits had values which resembled those of the ovariectomized rabbits. Hough and Zilversmit[8] demonstrated a 'dramatically' retarded development of arterial lesions in rabbits treated with intramuscular injections of 17β-estradiol cypionate as compared to control rabbits. This investigation is particularly interesting because it also suggested that the aortic influx of cholesteryl ester (nanogram of esterified cholesterol per milligram of aortic cholesterol per hour) was the same in estrogen-treated and untreated animals, whereas the per cent hydrolysis of newly entered cholesteryl ester was significantly lower in the estrogen-treated animals. Henriksson and colleagues[9] studied the influence of estradiol on atherogenesis and lipoprotein metabolism in male rabbits. Estradiol was given daily in the chow as well as in a weekly intramuscular injection. Their study demonstrated a significant anti-atherogenic effect of estradiol treatment.

The expression of the hepatic lipoprotein receptor was strongly suppressed by cholesterol feeding. This effect was counteracted by estrogen treatment and resulted in reduced plasma VLDL-cholesterol levels in estrogen-treated animals. These findings are in accordance with a study that demonstrated an estrogenic induction of mRNA for the hepatic LDL-receptor with increased LDL-receptor levels and a fall in plasma cholesterol levels as the outcome[10].

Recently, a study in 48 rabbits that used estradiol or progesterone or different dose combinations of the two suggested that the beneficial estradiol effect could be eliminated when it was combined with high progesterone doses, which produce continuously elevated 17OH-progesterone levels[11].

OUR STUDIES

Our initial study[12] included 75 cholesterol-fed rabbits. Fifteen rabbits had a sham operation,

whereas the remaining 60 were bilaterally ovariectomized and randomly assigned to receive either estrogen alone or estrogen in combination with either norethisterone acetate or levonorgestrel. The last ovari-ectomized group received placebo. This study strongly supported the anti-atherogenic effect of estradiol and indicated that a large part of this beneficial effect was not explained by a lowering effect on serum lipids and lipoproteins. This study also indicated that the continuous addition of two commonly prescribed 19-nortestosterone derivatives did not counteract the significant beneficial estrogenic effect.

Our next study using 60 cholesterol-fed rabbits further explored the anti-atherogenic effect of oral estrogen monotherapy and, in addition, evaluated the impact of continuous monotherapy with either norethisterone acetate or levonorgestrel[13]. The principal finding was that estradiol treatment had an anti-atherogenic effect equivalent to a 40% reduction in plasma total cholesterol (Figure

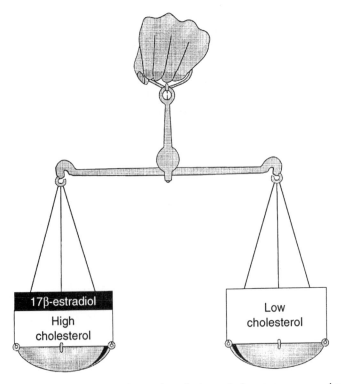

Figure 1 Estrogen treatment, in terms of atherosclerosis, is equivalent to an approximately 40% reduction in plasma total cholesterol

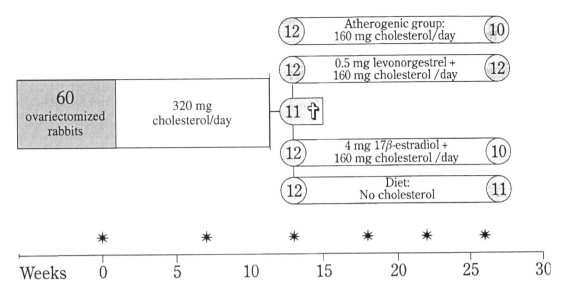

Figure 2 The design of the secondary prevention study. *Represents measurement of serum lipids and lipoproteins

1). Both progestogen groups had virtually the same degree of atherosclerosis as seen in the placebo group, supporting the neutral effect on atherogenesis found in our previous study[12].

The arterial uptake of LDL particles was then examined in 20 rabbits not fed cholesterol; these were randomly assigned to receive either 17β-estradiol or placebo[14]. After 10 weeks, the arterial permeability to LDL was measured using iodinated LDL particles. The aortic permeability to LDL was virtually identical in the two groups. This finding is thus in agreement with the study by Hough and Zilversmit[8] and supports the hypothesis that estrogens exert their direct effect on the intra-arterial metabolism of lipids rather than on the arterial uptake of these particles.

Recently, we evaluated the role of female sex hormones on established atherosclerosis induced by a 13-week cholesterol feeding period[15]. In week 14, the rabbits were assigned to four groups to receive a cholesterol-free diet, a moderately cholesterol enriched diet, a moderately cholesterol-enriched diet plus 17β-estradiol or levonorgestrel (Figure 2). This secondary prevention study showed that rabbits fed a moderately atherogenic diet plus estradiol tended to have less atherosclerosis than rabbits fed the cholesterol-free chow. The two groups which received a moderately atherogenic diet with or without oral levonorgestrel had virtually the same degree of atherosclerosis, which was approximately twice as much as in the estradiol group. Further analysis again indicated a direct anti-atherogenic effect of estradiol.

CONCLUSION

Results obtained with the cholesterol-fed rabbit model have consistently shown an anti-atherogenic effect of estrogen treatment, whereas most progestogens seem to have a neutral impact on atherogenesis. The estrogenic effect on atherogenesis is only partly explained by beneficial changes in plasma lipids. The available data indicate, furthermore, that estrogens have a favorable impact on the intra-arterial metabolism of cholesterol. Recent data obtained in rabbits suggest that the direct beneficial effect of estradiol is at least partly dependent on an intact endothelium[16,17].

References

1. Rosenfeld ME, Ross R. Macrophage and smooth muscle cell proliferation in atherosclerotic lesions of WHHL and comparably hypercholesterolemic fat-fed rabbits. *Arteriosclerosis* 1990;10:680–7

2. Armstrong ML, Heistad DD. Animal models of atherosclerosis. *Atherosclerosis* 1990;85:15–23

3. Constantinides P, Gutmann-Auersperg N, Hopes D, *et al.* Estriol and prednisolone in rabbit atherosclerosis. *Arch Pathol* 1962;73:277–80

4. Pick R, Stamler J, Rodbard S, *et al.* The inhibition of coronary atherosclerosis by estrogens in cholesterol-fed chicks. *Circulation* 1952;6:276–80

5. Souadjian JV, Kottke BA, Titus JL. Estrogen effect on spontaneous atherosclerosis. *Arch Path* 1968;85:463–7

6. Kushwaha RS, Hazzard WR. Exogenous estrogens attenuate dietary hypercholesterolemia and atherosclerosis in the rabbit. *Metabolism* 1981;30:359–66

7. Fischer GM, Swain ML. Effects of estradiol and progesterone on the increased synthesis of collagen in atherosclerotic rabbit aortas. *Atherosclerosis* 1985;54:177–85

8. Hough JL, Zilversmit DB. Effect of 17 beta estradiol on aortic cholesterol content and metabolism in cholesterol-fed rabbits. *Arteriosclerosis* 1986;6:57–63

9. Henriksson P, Stamberger M, Eriksson M, *et al.* Oestrogen-induced changes in lipoprotein metabolism: role in prevention of atherosclerosis in the cholesterol-fed rabbit. *Eur J Clin Invest* 1989;19:395–403

10. Ma PTS, Yamamoto T, Goldstein JL, *et al.* Increased mRNA for low density lipoprotein receptor in livers of rabbits treated with 17α-ethinyl estradiol. *Proc Natl Acad Sci USA* 1986;83:792–6

11. Hanke H, Hanke S, Bruck B, *et al.* Inhibition of the protective effect of estrogen by progesterone in experimental atherosclerosis. *Atherosclerosis* 1996;121:129–38

12. Haarbo J, Leth-Espensen P, Stender S, *et al.* Estrogen monotherapy and combined estrogen-progestogen replacement therapy attenuate aortic accumulation of cholesterol in ovariectomized cholesterol-fed rabbits. *J Clin Invest* 1991;87:1274–9

13. Haarbo J, Svendsen OL, Christiansen C. Progestogens do not affect aortic accumulation of cholesterol in ovariectomized cholesterol-fed rabbits. *Circ Res* 1992;70:1198–1202

14. Haarbo J, Nielsen LB, Stender S, *et al.* Aortic permeability to LDL during estrogen therapy. A study in normocholesterolemic rabbits. *Arterioscler Thromb* 1994;14:243–7

15. Haarbo J, Christiansen C. The impact of female sex hormones on secondary prevention of atherosclerosis in ovariectomized cholesterol-fed rabbits. *Atherosclerosis* 1996;123:139–44

16. Holm P, Andersen HO, Nordestgaard BG, *et al.* The effect of oestrogen replacement therapy on development of experimental arteriosclerosis: a study in transplanted and balloon-injured rabbit aortas. *Atherosclerosis* 1995;115:191–200

17. Holm P, Korsgaard N, Shalmi M, *et al.* Long-term inhibition of NO synthesis significantly reduces the antiatherogenic effect of estrogen in cholesterol-fed oophorectomized rabbits. Abstract presented at the *3rd Annual Scandinavian Atherosclerosis Conference*, Humlebaek, Denmark, 1996

The effect of sex steroids on cardiovascular risk factors

16

R. Sitruk-Ware

INTRODUCTION

It is now well-established that cardiovascular disease (CVD) represents the major cause of death in women just as in men, but at a later age. In women the incidence of CVD increases after the menopause and it has been shown that the risk of atherosclerosis increases by three- to four-fold after a natural menopause[1].

Furthermore, in the mid-1950s, autopsy studies showed that the prevalence of coronary stenosis was similar in women who had undergone oophorectomy and in men of the same age group.

A number of epidemiological studies performed since the early 1980s indicate an approximately 50% reduction in cardiovascular morbidity and mortality in women using estrogens after the menopause[2-4]. However, the controversy is ongoing as regards a possible selection bias in the studies; healthier women receive estrogens for long-term use more often than women at risk[4].

Recently, a better understanding of the mechanisms underlying the protective effect of estrogens was provided by animal studies using the monkey model[5] as well as studies of postmenopausal women, using surrogate markers of cardiovascular risk[6,7]. There is now evidence that estrogens will improve endothelial function and hence vascular tone, as well as improving the lipid profile[8], carbohydrate metabolism[9] and hemostatic parameters[10].

The controversy was raised again regarding the role of progestins, prescribed together with estrogens to protect the endometrium, and shown for some of the most prescribed molecules partially to oppose the beneficial effect of estrogens[11,12]. Unfortunately, that concern was directed towards progestins as a class effect, although several categories of progestins are often prescribed, and striking differences exist in the types of molecule that have been tested[13-15].

Obviously, natural progesterone and some of its derivatives such as the 19-norprogesterone molecules do not exert any androgenic effect[13,15] and hence no negative effect on the lipids, while the 19-nortesterone derivatives and even some 17-hydroxy-progesterone molecules exert a partial androgenic effect[13,16], explaining some of the negative effects observed on cardiovascular risk factors or surrogate markers of risk.

Given these class differences, it would be inappropriate to claim that progestins in general compromise the cardioprotective effects of estrogens without specifying which of these progestins reverse the estrogen effects and which do not, as indicated by the existing data.

RISK FACTORS FOR CARDIOVASCULAR DISEASE

Among the main cardiovascular risk factors recognized for both men and women, cigarette smoking, high cholesterol levels, hypertension, diabetes mellitus and obesity may be preventable causes of coronary heart disease[17].

In women, the estrogen deprivation following the menopause may affect several of these risk factors and it is now well accepted that estrogen replacement therapy (ERT) will improve cholesterol levels, diastolic blood pressure, insulin sensitivity and some of the clotting factors[8–10,13].

The existence of atherosclerosis in the vessel tree definitely increases the risk of cardiovascular disease. The beneficial effects of estrogens on the vasodilating endothelial factors, and hence on vasomotion[18], would play a major role in the primary prevention of coronary heart disease in women[17].

EFFECT OF ESTROGENS AND PROGESTINS ON THE CARDIOVASCULAR RISK FACTORS

Effects on lipids and lipoproteins

Lipid profile in postmenopausal women

Cross-sectional studies[8,19] and longitudinal studies[20] have indicated that menopause by itself will affect the lipid profile. Stevenson and colleagues[19] studied 542 women aged between 18 and 70 years and compared the lipid values of postmenopausal women with those of premenopausal women.

The most striking changes relate to the cholesterol bound to low-density lipoproteins (LDL-C) which increases up to 25% after the menopause and to the cholesterol bound to high-density lipoproteins (HDL-C), especially the HDL2 subfraction, which decreases by around 25%.

It was also reported that lipoprotein (a) increased after the menopause and the LDL particle size became smaller and denser[8].

Effects of estrogens

Most of the studies evaluating the effect of sex steroids on lipoproteins indicated a reduction of LDL-C levels and an increase of HDL-C levels by 10–15%[21].

Estrogen therapy, regardless of its type and route of administration, lowers total cholesterol and LDL-C and the effect is maintained for as long as the treatment is given[8,22]. It has also been shown that estrogen protects against lipoprotein oxidation, one major step in the atherogenic process, by increasing the lag time of oxidation[23].

The effect of estrogens on HDL-C varies according to the type, the dose and the route of administration of the steroid[8,24–27]. Also, the duration of the administration is important to consider, as indeed the variation of the lipoprotein is rapid after an oral intake due to the direct liver effect. In contrast, the change appears only after 24 weeks of administration with a non-oral route of application, as the liver is by-passed, and a steady state is usually obtained after 4–6 months for lipid metabolism.

The route of administration of estrogens is also important as far as triglycerides (TG) variations are concerned. Indeed, TGs increase by 15–20% with oral estrogens but decrease under percutaneous or transdermal estradiol by around 15%, this effect reflecting rather a physiological effect of estrogen[8,25,28].

Effects of the progestins

The addition of a progestin to ERT may affect the lipid formula, however the effects differ according to the type of the progestogen. Progestogens with androgenic properties partially reverse the HDL-raising effect of estrogen[8,13,29], while natural progesterone and some 19-norprogesterone derivatives such as nomegestrol acetate do not affect the HDL levels[13,30].

In the Postmenopausal Estrogen/Progestin Intervention Trial[13], the PEPI trial, 875 postmenopausal women were followed for 3 years in a randomized, double-blind, placebo-controlled trial.

The three combined regimens of estrogen and progestin induced an increase in HDL levels and a decrease in LDL levels. However, the increase in HDL-C was partially reversed in the groups in which medroxyprogesterone acetate (MPA) was added to oral estrogens while oral micronized progesterone did not modify the estrogen-induced rise. The results observed for LDL under estrogen were not modified by the addition of a progestin, either MPA or progesterone.

In the study of Crook and co-workers[29], in which 19-nortestosterone derivatives were evaluated in a 6-month randomized comparative study, levonorgestrel given orally significantly reversed the HDL-raising effect of estrogen. Norethisterone acetate (NETA) given transdermally in doses as low as 250 μg per day also reversed the estrogen effect, although to a lesser extent than was observed with levonorgestrel.

In another randomized, comparative, double-blind trial comparing the effects of nomegestrol acetate (NOM Ac) to NETA, both given orally at the dose of 5 mg/day, the increase in HDL-C observed under estradiol valerate was partially reversed by NETA but not by NOM Ac, a 19-norprogesterone derivative[30].

Moreover, in a 3-month randomized prospective study comparing the effect of a placebo and two oral estradiol + NOM Ac combinations, the progestin being given at doses of 2.5 and 3.75 mg daily for 14 days per cycle, NOM Ac did not reverse the effects of oral estradiol on LDL-C and apolipoprotein A_1. It also induced a significant decrease in lipoprotein (a), as was previously observed with MPA[31].

These results indicate that it is not the dose or route of administration that is the most important factor to consider for the effect of progestins on HDL, but rather the molecule from which they derive. Those progestogens derived from progesterone and devoid of androgenic properties do not impede the beneficial estrogenic effects.

Role of lipid changes in cardiovascular risk

The relevance of these lipid changes has to be questioned. First of all, the role of HDL changes in the alleged cardiovascular protective effects of estrogens accounts for 30 to a maximum of 50% of these effects[31]. Also, in an epidemiological study analyzing the relative risk of myocardial infarction of estrogen–progestin users versus non-users, a 'protective' effect appeared for all therapies as compared to no treatment, even in the group using levonorgestrel, the most androgenic of the progestins used so far in hormone replacement therapy (HRT)[32].

In the 15 August, 1996, issue of the *New England Journal of Medicine*, Grodstein and colleagues[33] reported the relationship between cardiovascular disease and HRT in 59 337 women followed for up to 16 years. Compared with the risk of major coronary heart disease for women who did not use hormones, the relative risk was 0.6 for women using estrogens alone and even lower at 0.39 for those using combined hormones. The authors found no association between stroke and use of combined hormones. For this study, conducted in the USA, the progestin used was most likely medroxyprogesterone acetate.

Although this large observational study confirms the previous results of Falkeborn and colleagues[34] in Sweden and Psaty and associates[35] in the USA, the possibility of a selection bias is raised again. Women who stay on long-term HRT are usually healthier on average than those who do not, with lower blood pressure and lower weight and they exercise more often. Grodstein and co-workers[33] have adjusted for these confounding factors, as did the other researchers. However, only the long-term randomized controlled trial of the Women's Health Initiative will bring a definite conclusion.

Before then, as a practical recommendation, one should conclude that, overall, the effects of most HRT treatments on lipids and lipoproteins would seem to be on balance beneficial[8], but the selection of the least androgenic progestins should be recommended for long-term therapy.

Effects of estrogens and progestins on carbohydrate metabolism

Glucose intolerance and hyperinsulinemia are well-known risk factors for cardiovascular disease. Postmenopausal women have an age-related deterioration of glucose metabolism[36] and have been shown to have a reduced number of peripheral insulin receptors compared with premenopausal women in the early follicular phase[37].

Insulin is a potent stimulus to endothelial cell growth and also regulates LDL receptor activity[38,39]. Therefore, a reduction in fasting insulin levels may be important in controlling one of the mechanisms of CVD.

De Cleyn and co-workers[40] conducted an 8-month study in which 20 women received 0.625 mg conjugated equine estrogens per day, given alone for 2 months, then with the addition of dydrogesterone 20 mg/day for 12 days per month for the following 6 months. Oral glucose tolerance tests (OGTT) performed before and after each treatment regimen showed a decrease in the area under the glycemia curve with both treatments. A slight increase in insulinemia was found in the combined treatment group but was not statistically significant.

Cagnacci and associates[41] using transdermal estradiol therapy showed a reduction in fasting insulin levels and an increased hepatic insulin clearance suggesting a beneficial effect of estradiol on glucose metabolism when given transdermally.

Later, Godsland and colleagues[9], in an open, randomized comparative study of 61 postmenopausal women, evaluated the effect of oral equine estrogens with sequential oral levonorgestrel (0.075 mg/day, 12 days/month) or transdermal estradiol with sequential transdermal NETA (0.250 mg/day, 14 days/month). Using intravenous glucose tolerance tests they found that oral therapy caused a deterioration of glucose tolerance and an overall increase in plasma insulin, most probably due to the androgenic properties of norgestrel. On the other hand, no change in insulin response or in glucose occurred with the transdermal therapy although the progestin used also exhibited some androgenic effects on lipids[29] but obviously did not affect carbohydrate metabolism when given transdermally.

The 19-norprogesterone derivatives appear to be neutral towards the carbohydrate metabolism, as shown by Dorangeon and co-workers[42], studying the nomegestrol acetate effect in premenopausal women. In these women who did not receive exogenous estrogens, the administration of NOM Ac at doses of 5 mg/day over 20 days per cycle for 6 months did not affect the response in plasma glucose and plasma insulin in the OGTT.

Estrogen and progestin effects on the hemostatic risk factors for cardiovascular disease

The suggested preventive effect of sex steroids on the development of atherosclerosis might be counteracted by their possible thrombogenic effect indicated by recent studies among oral contraceptive users. Obviously ethinyl estradiol contained in the contraceptive pill is no longer used in ERT and the so-called third generation progestins are not yet widely used for HRT.

In the large cohort studies and essentially the Nurses' Health Study[33] no significant association has ever been found between stroke and hormones. In a recent observational study[43] current users of HRT have been found to be at increased risk of venous thromboembolism. The risk seems to be restricted to the first year of therapy. In that study the risk was similar in both oral estrogen users and transdermal estrogen users[43]. The fact that the risk appears to be concentrated in the first year would suggest that some women, more sensitive or with predisposing factors, would develop thrombotic events with any ERT and then stop therapy, while the other women who tolerate it better remain in the longer-term users' group. Therefore, it is of the utmost importance to investigate the effects of the various sex steroids on hemostatic parameters in order to select for therapy those devoid of unwanted effects.

In the large 3-year PEPI trial already mentioned, the combined regimen of equine estrogens plus MPA or plus progesterone lowered fibrinogen levels[13], one of the markers considered to be an independent risk factor for myocardial infarction and stroke[10].

The plasma fibrinogen concentrations increase with age, especially during the menopausal transition. In a recent 2-year open prospective study, 42 postmenopausal women received estradiol given transdermally (50 μg/day) and MPA (5 mg/day, 12 days every second month). The hemostatic risk factors were measured at baseline, at 3 months and after 2 years of treatment and compared to the results observed in an untreated control group of 18 postmenopausal women as well as a reference group of 20 premenopausal women.

Fibrinogen levels significantly decreased under HRT while it slightly increased in the untreated women. Similarly, FVII antigen and PAI-1 antigen decreased after 2 years of treatment, but slightly increased in the control group. There were no changes in antithrombin III or protein C values in any group. Therefore, a beneficial effect of the sex steroids used in the study was demonstrated on the hemostatic parameters involved, as a defense system against thrombosis[10].

In previous studies using transdermal estradiol, both short- and long-term, no effects on the hemostasis variables were found[28]. Also, with a progestin other than MPA, Basdevant and colleagues[44] showed no effect of nomegestrol acetate on plasminogen, fibrinogen, or proteins C and S. The only change observed was a significant increase in antithrombin III which indeed is not a negative effect.

Effects of estrogens and progesterone on blood pressure

There are some discrepancies in the literature regarding estrogen therapy and blood pressure: some authors report an increase in blood pressure in a small percentage of oral estrogen users and others report no change or a decrease in systolic blood pressure[45]. The different results may be related to the variety of therapeutic regimens that constitute ERT.

Recently, Foidart and co-workers[46] have evaluated the effect of transdermal estradiol (50 μg/day) on the blood pressure of hypertensive women whose condition was therapeutically controlled. Only one patient out of 92 experienced an increase in diastolic blood pressure; no effect of transdermal estradiol was detected on either the systolic or diastolic blood pressure of the remaining 91 patients. Long-term treatment with a combined regimen of transdermal estradiol and MPA in normotensive postmenopausal women was reported by Pang and colleagues[47]. In this case, treatment was associated with a reduction in mean systolic and diastolic blood pressures.

Oral estrogens have been shown to increase renin substrate in a dose-dependent manner. However, earlier studies, compared with later studies, may reflect the prescription of higher doses of estrogen by doctors. For example, Chetkowski and co-workers[48] reported no change in renin substrate with a low dose of equine estrogens or with transdermal estradiol. Moreover, long-term therapy with non-oral estrogens has been shown to maintain blood pressure in the normal range[49]. The effect of a high dose of potent oral estrogens on renin substrate may explain some of the earlier findings of an increased prevalence of hypertension in estrogen users[50].

However, other mechanisms of action of estrogen on blood vessels must be taken into consideration. Estrogens appear to stimulate the production of prostacylin within the arterial endothelial cells, which induces a vasodilating effect and a consequent fall in blood pressure. On the other hand, the stimulation of angiotensin production by estrogens exerts a vasospastic effect on the vasculature through stimulation of thromboxane production. A balance between these two opposing effects may occur in the vessels, and may explain why only a small percentage of women develop an increase in blood pressure. It has been hypothesized that a protective mechanism exists which counteracts the vasospastic effect of angiotensin; according to this hypothesis, this mechanism is probably due to the influence of estrogens[50].

Effects of estrogens and progestins on vessels

Effect of estrogens on the vascular wall

The most recent studies regarding the mechanisms by which estrogens may afford cardioprotective effects have examined their effect on the vessels, and especially on endothelial function. The presence of estrogen binding sites in endothelial cells has been documented in animal and human arteries[51]. A direct effect of estrogens on the endothelium has been suggested and may be related to the binding of the steroids to their receptors.

The endothelium is actively involved in regulating vascular tone through the production of endothelial factors with vasodilating or vasoconstricting properties[6]. Hayashi and associates[52] have found evidence of a greater production of nitric oxide in the female, rather than the male, rabbit aorta, suggesting that estrogens might affect the release of this endothelial vasodilating factor.

Rosselli and co-workers[53], investigating postmenopausal women, measured serum levels of nitrite/nitrate ($NO_2 + NO_3$) at regular intervals over 24 months. The levels remained unchanged in the untreated women but increased significantly in a treated group of 31 women receiving a combination of transdermal estradiol and oral norethisterone acetate. The increase was statistically significant in the samples taken during the estrogen-only phase and not in the samples taken during the progestin phase, suggesting that NETA counteracted the estrogen-related increase of NO. Given the technical difficulties of measuring NO in blood samples, similar studies in women have not been repeated.

Foidart and colleagues[54] have documented the increased production of prostacyclin metabolites in postmenopausal women treated with percutaneous estradiol, but not with oral estrogen. Prostacyclin exerted a vasodilatory action on the blood vessels while thromboxane, also produced by the endothelium, induced vasoconstriction. Estrogens appear to regulate the balance between vasodilatory and vasoconstrictive factors, favoring the vasodilatation effect.

In the cynomolgus monkey[5,18], it was shown that 17β-estradiol modulated the responses of the coronary arteries of the animals to acetylcholine (ACh). Estrogen-deprived atherosclerotic monkeys were compared to animals receiving estrogen replacement therapy. The degree of coronary artery constriction following an infusion of ACh was measured in both groups of animals. Paradoxical vasoconstriction occurred following ACh in the untreated animals while estradiol therapy restored the normal endothelium-dependent vasodilatation. The process occurred rapidly, vasomotion being restored to normal within 20 min of an intravenous injection of estrogens.

Similar regulation of vasomotion was found in women with coronary disease, those receiving ERT exhibiting a dose-dependent vasodilation in response to ACh, in contrast with the untreated women who exhibited a vasoconstriction[55]. The changes observed in the vasomotion of the postmenopausal women appear to be as prompt as observed in monkeys[56].

More recently, Collins and colleagues[57] showed that intracoronary estradiol decreased the ACh-induced vasoconstriction in nine postmenopausal women, but not in seven men of similar age. It has also been shown by the same authors that 17β-estradiol exerts calcium antagonist properties[58]. Therefore, its protective effects against atherosclerotic disease may involve the same mechanism as that of calcium channel blockers, which have been shown to have a beneficial effect on the development of early atheromatous lesions.

Effects of progestins on the vascular wall

It has been suggested that progestins would partially reverse the estrogenic effects, on the assumption that these molecules exert an anti-estrogenic effect at several target levels.

Sullivan and colleagues[11] studied the effects of conjugated equine estrogens given alone during 21 days and with added progestin, MPA

10 mg for 10 days, on forearm vascular resistance in postmenopausal women. They found that resting vascular resistance and resistance after cold pressor stimulation rose significantly and at a higher level during combined treatment than after estrogen alone.

In the monkey model, as described above[11], the addition of cyclic or continuous MPA to estrogens inhibited ACh responses by 50%[59].

These findings raised a potentially harmful effect of some progestins such as MPA in postmenopausal women. Other progestins devoid of androgenic effects are being tested and results are expected soon.

CONCLUSION

It has been shown that 17β-estradiol decreases the extent of atheroma in monkeys, stimulates the release of endothelial vasodilator factors in the rabbit aorta, and favors vessel relaxation by other non-endothelium-related mechanisms. In humans, an increase in the production of prostacyclin metabolites with estradiol therapy has been reported.

In addition, the major parameters involved in chronic cardiovascular risk, VLDL, LDL-cholesterol, hyperinsulinemia and hypertension, have been shown to be favorably influenced by estrogens, including transdermal estradiol. These effects tend to suggest that oral and non-oral administration of estradiol have a favorable influence on cardiovascular risk, but further studies are needed to confirm this trend. Epidemiological studies provide only part of the documentation of the beneficial effect of estrogens. Additional studies that demonstrate a favorable influence of estrogen on all risk factors for cardiovascular disease in women should be considered.

Also, the role of various progestins should be documented further. It appears that, although some progestins with androgenic properties partially reverse the estrogenic effects on lipids and vasomotion, other molecules without any androgenic property do not reverse the beneficial effect of estrogens on the CVD risk markers.

References

1. Wittemen J, Grobbee D, Kof F, et al. Increased risk of atherosclerosis in women after the menopause. Br Med J 1989;298:642–4
2. Stampfer MJ, Colditz GA. Estrogen replacement therapy and coronary heart disease: a quantitative assessment of the epidemiologic evidence. Prev Med 1991;20:47–63
3. Grady D, Rubin SM, Petitti DB, et al. Hormone therapy to prevent disease and prolong life in postmenopausal women. Ann Intern Med 1992; 117:1016–37
4. Meade T, Berra A. Hormone replacement therapy and cardiovascular disease. Br Med Bull 1992;48/2:276–308
5. Clarkson TB, Anthony MS, Potvin Klein K. Hormone replacement therapy and coronary artery atherosclerosis: the monkey model. Br J Obstet Gynecol 1996;103(S13):53–8
6. Sullivan JM. Hormone replacement therapy and cardiovascular disease: the human model. Br J Obstet Gynecol 1996;103(S13):59–67
7. Holdright DR, Sullivan AK, Wright CA, et al. Acute effect of estrogen replacement therapy on treadmill performance in postmenopausal women with coronary artery disease. Eur Heart J 1995;16:1566–70
8. Stevenson JC. Are changes in lipoproteins during HRT important? Br J Obstet Gynecol 1996; 103(S13):39–44
9. Godsland IF, Gangar K, Walton C, et al. Insulin resistance, secretion, and elimination in postmenopausal women receiving oral or transdermal hormone replacement therapy. Metabolism 1993;42:846–53
10. Lindoff C, Peterson F, Lecander I, et al. Transdermal estrogen replacement therapy: beneficial effects on hemostatic risk factors for cardiovascular disease. Maturitas 1996;24:43–50
11. Sullivan JM, Shala LA, Miller LA, et al. Progestin enhances vasoconstrictor responses in postmenopausal women receiving estrogen replacement therapy. Menopause 1995;2:193–9

12. Clarkson TB. *HRT and CVD: The Monkey Model.* Presented at the 10th International Congress of Endocrinology, June 12–15, 1996, San Francisco, USA. Abstract book, Vol 1(S9-1);25

13. The Writing Group for the PEPI Trial. Effects of estrogen or estrogen/progestin regimens on heart disease risk factors in postmenopausal women: The Postmenopausal Estrogen/Progestin Interventions (PEPI) Trial. *J Am Med Assoc* 1995;273:199–208

14. Adams MR, Kaplan JR, Manuck SB, *et al.* Inhibition of coronary artery atherosclerosis by 17β-estradiol in ovariectomised monkeys. Lack of an effect of added progesterone. *Arteriosclerosis* 1990;10:1051–7

15. Duc I, Botella J, Bonnet P, *et al.* Antiandrogenic properties of nomegestrol acetate. *Arzneim Forsch/Drug Res* 1995;45:70–7

16. Bradley DD, Wingerd J, Petitti DB, *et al.* Serum high-density-lipoprotein cholesterol in women using oral contraceptives, estrogens and progestins. *N Engl J Med* 1978;299:17–20

17. Rich-Edwards JW, Mason JE, Hennekens CH, *et al.* The primary prevention of coronary heart disease in women. *N Engl J Med* 1995;332:1758–66

18. Williams JK, Adams MR, Klopfenstein HS. Estrogen modulates responses of atherosclerotic coronary arteries. *Circulation* 1990;81:1680–7

19. Stevenson JC, Crook D, Godsland IF. Influence of age and menopause on serum lipids and lipoproteins in healthy women. *Atherosclerosis* 1993;98:83–90

20. Matthews KA, Meilahn E, Kuller LH, *et al.* Menopause and risk factors for coronary heart disease. *N Engl J Med* 1989;321:641–6

21. Bush TL, Miller VT. Effects of pharmacologic agents used during menopause: impact on lipids and lipoproteins. In *Menopause Physiology and Pharmacology*, Mishell, Jr, ed. New York: Year Book Medical Publishers Inc., 1987;187–208

22. Whitcroft SI, Crook D, Marsh MS, *et al.* Long term effects of oral and transdermal hormone replacement therapies on serum lipid and lipoprotein concentrations. *Obstet Gynecol* 1994;84:222–6

23. Sack MN, Rader DJ, Cannon RO. Oestrogen and inhibition of oxidation of low-density lipoproteins in postmenopausal women. *Lancet* 1994;343:269–70

24. Samsioe G. Lipid profiles in estrogen users. Is there a key marker for the risk of cardiovasular disease. In Sitruk-Ware R, Utian WH, eds. *The Menopause and Hormonal Replacement Therapy. Facts and Controversies.* New York: Marcel Dekker Inc., 1991;181–200

25. Sitruk-Ware R, Ibarra de Palacios P. Oestrogen replacement therapy and cardiovascular disease in postmenopausal women. A review. *Maturitas* 1989;11:259–74

26. Stanczyk FZ, Shoupe D, Nunez V, *et al.* A randomized comparison of non oral estradiol delivery in postmenopausal women. *Am J Obstet Gynecol* 1988;159:1540–6

27. Jensen J, Riis BJ, Strom V, *et al.* Long term effects of percutaneous estrogens and oral progesterone on serum lipoproteins in postmenopausal women. *Am J Obstet Gynecol* 1987;156:66–71

28. Cheang A, Sitruk-Ware R, Samsioe G. Transdermal oestradiol and cardiovascular risk factors. *Br J Obstet Gynecol* 1994;101:571–81

29. Crook D, Cust MP, Gangar KF, *et al.* Comparison of transdermal and oral estrogen-progestin replacement therapy: effects on serum lipids and lipoproteins. *Am J Obstet Gynecol* 1992;166:950–5

30. Dorangeon P, Thomas JL, Gillery P. Short term effects on lipids and lipoproteins of two progestogens used in postmenopausal replacement therapy. *Eur J Clin Res* 1992;3:187–93

31. Conard J, Basdevant A, Thomas JL, *et al.* Cardiovascular risk factors and combined estrogen-progestin replacement therapy: a placebo-controlled study with nomegestrol acetate and estradiol. *Fertil Steril* 1995;64:957–62

32. Bush TL, Barrett-Connor E, Cowan LD, *et al.* Cardiovascular mortality and noncontraceptive use of estrogen in women: results from the Lipid Research Clinics Program follow-up study. *Circulation* 1987;75:1102–9

33. Grodstein F, Stampfer MJ, Manson JE, *et al.* Postmenopausal estrogen and progestin use and the risk of cardiovascular disease. *N Engl J Med* 1996;353:453–61

34. Falkeborn M, Persson I, Adami HO, *et al.* The risk of acute myocardial infarction after oestrogen and oestrogen-progestogen replacement. *Br J Obstet Gynaecol* 1992;99:821–8

35. Psaty BM, Heckbert SR, Atkins D, *et al.* The risk of myocardial infarction associated with the combined use of estrogens and progestins in postmenopausal women. *Arch Intern Med* 1994;154:1333–9

36. Jackson RA. Mechanisms of age-related glucose intolerance. *Diabetes Care* 1990;13(S2):9–19

37. De Pirro R, Fusco A, Bertoli A, *et al.* Insulin receptors during the menstrual cycle in normal women. *J Clin Endocrinol Metab* 1978;47:1387–9

38. Stout RW, Bierman EL, Ross R. Effect of insulin on the proliferation of cultured primate arterial smooth muscle cells. *Circ Res* 1975;36:319–27

39. Chait A, Bierman EL, Albers JJ. Low density lipoprotein receptor activity in cultured human skin fibroblasts. Mechanisms of insulin-induced stimulation. *J Clin Invest* 1979;64:1309–19

40. De Cleyn K, Buytaert P, Coppens M. Carbohydrate metabolism during hormonal substitution therapy. *Maturitas* 1989;11:235–42

41. Cagnacci A, Soldani R, Carriero PL, *et al.* Effects of low doses of transdermal 17β-estradiol on

carbohydrate metabolism in postmenopausal women. *J Clin Endocrinol Metab* 1992;74:1396–400

42. Dorangeon P, Thomas JL, Lumbroso M, *et al.* Effects of nomegestrol acetate on carbohydrate metabolism in premenopausal women. Presented at *XIII World Congress of Gynecology and Obstetrics* (Figo), Singapore, 1991, Abstract No 0636

43. Perez-Gutthann S, Garcia-Rodriguez LA, Duque-Oliart A, *et al.* HRT and the risk of venous thromboembolic event. *Pharmacoepidem Drug Safety* 1995;4(S1): Abstract 118,S53

44. Basdevant A, Pelissier C, Conrad J, *et al.* Effects of Nomegestrol Acetate (5mg/d) on hormonal, metabolic and hemostatic parameters in premenopausal women. *Contraception* 1991;44: 599–605

45. Sitruk-Ware R. Do estrogens protect against cardiovascular disease? In *The Menopause and Hormone Replacement Therapy. Facts and Controversies.* Sitruk-Ware R, Utian WH, eds. New York: Marcel Dekker, 1991;161–79

46. Foidart JM, Legrand JM, Van der Pas H, *et al.* The effects of estraderm TTS 50 + medroxy-progesterone acetate on blood pressure in hypertensive post-menopausal women. Unpublished

47. Pang SC, Green Dale GA, Cedars MI, *et al.* Long term effects of transdermal estradiol with and without medroxyprogesterone acetate. *Fertil Steril* 1993;59:76–82

48. Chetkowski RJ, Meldrum DR, Steingold KA, *et al.* Biologic effects of transdermal estradiol. *N Engl J Med* 1986;314:1615–20

49. Hassager C, Riis BJ, Strom V, *et al.* The long term effect of oral and percutaneous estradiol on plasma renin substrate and blood pressure. *Circulation* 1987;76:753–8

50. Wren BG. Hypertension and thrombosis with postmenopausal estrogen therapy. In Studd JWW. Whitehead MI, eds. *The Menopause.* London: Blackwell Scientific, 1988;181–9

51. Padwick ML, Whitehead MI, Coffer A, *et al.* Demonstration of an estrogen receptor-related protein in female tissues. In Studd JWW, Whitehead MI, eds. *The Menopause.* Oxford: Blackwell Scientific, 1988;227–33

52. Hayashi T, Fukoto JM, Ignarro LJ, *et al.* Basal release of nitric oxide from aortic rings is greater in female rabbits than in male rabbits: implications for atherosclerosis. *Proc Natl Acad Sci* 1992;89:11259–63

53. Rosselli M, Imthurn B, Keller PJ, *et al.* Circulating nitric oxide (nitrite/nitrite) levels in post-menopausal women substituted with 17β-estradiol and norethisterone acetate. A two-year follow-up study. *Hypertension* 1995;25(Part 2):848–53

54. Foidart JM, Dombrowicz N, de Lignières B. Urinary excretion of prostacylin and thromboxane metabolites in postmenopausal women treated with percutaneous estradiol (Ostrogel) or conjugated estrogens (Premarin®). In Dusitsin N, *et al.,* eds. *Physiological Hormone Replacement Therapy.* Carnforth: Parthenon Publishing, 1991:99–107

55. Herrington DM, Braden GA, Williams JK, *et al.* Endothelial-dependent coronary vasomotor responsiveness in postmenopausal women with and without estrogen replacement therapy. *Am J Cardiol* 1994;73:951–2

56. Rosano GMC, Sarrel PM, Poole-Wilson PA, *et al.* Beneficial effects of estrogen on exercise-induced myocardial ischaemia in women with coronary artery disease. *Lancet* 1993;342:133–6

57. Collins P, Rosano GMC, Sarrel PM, *et al.* 17β-Estradiol attenuates acetylcholine induced coronary arterial constriction in women but not men with coronary heart disease. *Circulation* 1995;92:24–30

58. Collins P, Rosano GMC, Jiang C, *et al.* Cardio-vascular protection by estrogen – a calcium antagonist effect. *Lancet* 1993;341:1264–6

59. Williams JK, Honoré EK, Washburn SA, *et al.* Effects of hormone replacement therapy on reactivity of atherosclerotic coronary arteries in cynomolgus monkeys. *J Am Coll Cardiol* 1994;24: 1757–61

New markers for cardiovascular diseases: intima-media thickness and compliance

17

M. Massonneau and A. Linhart

The assessment of cardiovascular risk in postmenopausal women is a subject involving various difficulties. Available epidemiological data, based on traditional surveys of cardiovascular risk factors in large populations, such as the Framingham Heart Study, were obtained before hormonal substitution was introduced in current practice. Cohort studies providing evidence of benefits of such treatment do not allow a reliable cardiovascular risk prediction, as their data are difficult to extrapolate to a general population sample. Furthermore, many confusing factors, such as an uneven time of onset, duration, composition and dosing of the replacement treatment, are difficult to take into account in current routine. Therefore, new, independent markers associated with the risk of cardiovascular morbidity and mortality are needed.

Arterial wall thickness is a useful parameter. Carotid intima-media thickening and early carotid atheroma were shown to be associated with a larger extent of coronary atherosclerosis and with higher cardiovascular morbidity. New computer-assisted techniques based on currently used two-dimensional vascular echography are allowing precise measurements of intima-media thickness to be made, that are easy to perform and highly reproducible. These systems are based on observer-independent algorithms analyzing changes in gray-level gradients. A recently developed system of anatomical masking further increases the reproducibility and facilitates long-term follow-up. Furthermore, this system improves the assessment of early atheroma progression or regression. Until recently, various sophisticated and costly systems used for determination of vascular distensibility were reserved for highly specialized laboratories. However, new technical developments in computer-assisted echography now allow the use of standard echographic equipment to acquire the data. Vascular distension represents a fundamental function necessary for arterial compliance assessment. This was shown to be related to atherosclerosis, traditional cardiovascular risk factors and left ventricular hypertrophy, probably reflecting a summation of influences of risk factors on the vessel wall over time.

The development of new, computer-assisted echography now allows assessments to be made of various markers, such as early atheroma, intima-media thickening and changes in vessel wall compliance. These parameters may be clinically relevant surrogates of cardiovascular morbidity which may be advantageously used for the assessment and follow-up of the protective role of hormone replacement treatment.

Monitoring of HRT for optimal cardiovascular protection

18

B. de Lignieres

Most publications advocate a larger use of hormone replacement therapy (HRT) in the prevention of cardiovascular diseases in postmenopausal women. However, because no randomized study is available, the exact magnitude of the potential vascular protection is unknown and the optimal indication, type, dose and route of administration of steroids are still undetermined. A 50% decrease in relative risk of almost all vascular events has been enthusiastically promised to all HRT users, especially to those at high risk, but more experts today conclude that no data are strong enough to support this claim[1-5]. HRT current users involved in the largest observational studies are likely to have been healthier than never users before starting the treatment, according to the prescribing practices of physicians[1-4]. They are also likely to have been selected through their lowest incidence of side effects and adverse events during treatment, in comparison with past users[2]. In similar circumstances, the compliance with a placebo has been shown to select the subjects with 50% less vascular morbidity and mortality than non-compliers[6]. Moreover, the most prescribed estrogen formulation does not achieve the expected goals even in a selected population. Some recent surveys, comparing the relatively small group of current users to the large group of never and past users or to estriol users (estriol is almost a placebo) do not find a significant decrease in the risk of coronary events[7-9], but a significant increase in deep vein thrombosis[10], pulmonary embolism[11] and also transient and ischemic strokes[12,13].

Additionally, the use of one of the most popular formulations of synthetic progestin has recently been suspected of annihilating the expected benefits of estrogens within the artery wall[14].

Furthermore, the current HRT prescriptions may not be optimal for all individuals and are still not approved for prevention of vascular diseases. Whether different steroids, doses, schedules and routes of administration with different metabolic consequences are preferable in some cases remains debatable, but no long-term comparative study is expected to be available soon. Any possibility of predicting the efficacy/safety ratio of a specific HRT preparation in any given individual is highly desirable, especially for smokers, obese women, dyslipidemics, diabetics, women over 60 years and those who are hypertensive or have a history of thromboembolism, all subjects for whom the right choice is crucial.

PLASMA LIPIDS

The first explanation for the protective effect of estradiol on cardiovascular diseases has been its influence on plasma lipids, specifically on high-density lipoprotein (HDL)-cholesterol[15]. In several studies, HDL-cholesterol levels were demonstrated to be a strong negative independent predictor of coronary disease in women, including postmenopausal women. Besides age, HDL-cholesterol is the most powerful predictor of death from cardiovascular causes in women with total cholesterol levels of less than 260 mg/dl, i.e. the majority of women of all ages.

However, measurement of plasma lipid changes does not seem to predict the vascular benefits and risks related to endogenous or exogenous estrogens and progestins. Before menopause, the ovarian secretion of sex steroids has a highly favorable influence on vascular risks, independently of cholesterol levels[16].

After menopause, the rapid rise in cardiovascular morbidity and mortality has no correlation with any change in plasma lipoproteins, especially with HDL changes, which are quite slow and limited[17,18]. In an experimental primate model, castration and substitution with various estrogens combined or not with progestins had a striking influence on coronary vasomotion and the atherosclerosis process, but again without any significant correlation with plasma lipoprotein changes[14].

Even the large variations of HDL-cholesterol induced by oral estrogens or progestins with a pharmacological liver first-pass effect had no visible influence on an experimental atherosclerosis model that may be explained by their specific mechanism of action.

In untreated pre- and postmenopausal women, HDL-cholesterol and triglyceride variation are strongly inversely related[19], suggesting a predominant physiological control by lipoprotein lipase. This enzyme, located mainly in muscle and adipose tissue, is primarily responsible for the degradation of very low-density lipoprotein (VLDL). During this process, the smaller and denser HDL particles called HDL_3 receive the fractions of cholesterol and phospholipids released from lipolyzed VLDL and also from peripheral cells with high cholesterol content (such as injured intima), and become larger and less dense HDL_2 particles. The most visible consequences of high lipoprotein lipase activity are low total triglycerides and high HDL_2-cholesterol plasma levels[20], which are expected to ensure the reverse transport of cholesterol from peripheral tissues to liver cells for clearance and metabolism. Lifestyle factors, such as cessation of cigarette smoking,

physical exercise, weight loss and carbohydrate metabolism improvement have been shown to increase HDL-cholesterol and decrease coronary artery events in men and, to a lesser extent, in women. In all of these situations, a rise in HDL-cholesterol coincides with a drop in triglycerides, primarily related to lipoprotein lipase activation[21]. Drugs proven effective in raising HDL-cholesterol and decreasing the incidence of coronary events also decrease triglycerides and are thought to act through lipoprotein lipase activation[21].

On the other hand, oral estrogens induce a parallel increase in HDL_2-cholesterol and triglycerides by a different mechanism – a decrease in hepatic lipase activity[22,23]. This mechanism tends to induce an accumulation of free cholesterol, phospholipids and triglycerides within the HDL particles by decreasing their hepatic clearance. There is no available evidence that this specific mechanism, which may not improve the reverse transport of cholesterol, has any beneficial consequences in animals, men or women[21]. Therefore, the quite limited rise in HDL-cholesterol measured after a few years of HRT and associated with a marked increase in triglycerides[24] cannot be taken as a reliable predictor of potential improvement in vascular risk.

In the same way, oral estrogens induce a fast decrease in LDL-cholesterol, which is expected to be beneficial. However, because the ratio of apoprotein B to LDL-cholesterol increases, creating smaller and denser particles that are theoretically more atherogenic[21,25], the actual benefit is unclear[26,27]. Significant LDL-cholesterol plasma changes during oral estrogen treatments have no predictive value in experimental studies[14].

The cholesterol transfer from circulating LDL particles to intima through macrophages and the subsequent cholesterol accumulation in the arterial wall are dramatically reduced by the physiological plasma concentration of estradiol[28]. The very early effect of HRT seems to be the reduction by 70–90% of regional degradation of LDL particles by the arterial wall, specifically in coronary arteries and carotid bifurcations.

This effect is measurable before the development of grossly visible artherosclerotic lesions and intimal thickening. It is localized in specific arterial sites, being more active in coronary than in cerebral arteries, and does not imply a significant reduction of LDL metabolism at other extra-arterial sites such as the liver, adrenal gland, spleen, kidney, intestine, skin and muscle.

Therefore, estradiol does not rapidly change the plasma values of LDL-cholesterol nor the whole body fractional catabolic rate of LDL, but locally protects some limited specific areas of the arterial tree by decreasing the high rate of LDL degradation responsible for cholesterol accumulation in arterial intima. Estradiol does not act as a lipid-lowering drug, as does niacin or gemfibrozil, but as a drug decreasing LDL oxidation and captation by macrophages. However, the predictive value of the measurement of LDL oxidation has not been validated and this is not available as a routine test.

Triglycerides tend to increase slowly after menopause but quite rapidly during oral estrogen treatment[24]. Because this fast and sustained change is observed exclusively with oral estrogens but not during non-oral administration of estradiol[26], the rise in triglycerides is likely to measure the intensity of the liver first-pass effect and to be correlated with other hepatic pharmacological changes such as coagulation factors[29].

In this case the rise in triglycerides should not be interpreted as a classical predictor of insulin resistance and fibrinolysis impairment, but mostly as a warning, indicating a potential hemostasis disturbance of liver origin[30].

OTHER RISK FACTORS

None of the other classical risk factors has been found to be consistently associated with the cardioprotective effect of estrogens or to be able to predict the vascular consequences of estrogen deprivation.

Before menopause, even women exposed to high blood pressure, obesity, tabagism and stress benefit from a strong protection in comparison with men[16]. During the menopause transition, no significant change in weight and blood pressure precede the increase in vascular relative risk[17,18]. Also, intervention studies do not indicate that substantial benefits can be expected from changes in weight, blood pressure or insulin resistance in treated postmenopausal women[24]. Therefore, HRT cannot be monitored by these measurements, even if most investigators recommend stopping or at least modifying the HRT in patients with rapid increase in weight, blood pressure or insulin resistance.

More useful information may be obtained by measurements of body composition instead of body mass index, or adaptation of blood pressure and heart rate to stress and exercise[31] instead of blood pressure at rest, but the appropriate methodologies are likely to be too expensive and too complex for routine monitoring.

VASOMOTION

One important part of the vascular benefits expected from HRT is the re-establishment of the physiological vasoactive responses to ischemia, exercise or cold.

The methodology for measuring vasodilatation in the forearm after a standardized ischemic or cold test is precise enough to differentiate optimal and insufficient circulating levels of estradiol and also optimal and suboptimal progestin effects[32,33].

The vasodilating effect of estrogens is likely to be at least partly related to nitric oxide activity. Both vasodilatation and plasma levels of nitric oxide are correlated with circulating levels of estrogens. As during the menstrual cycle, estradiol plasma levels of less than 80 pg/ml during replacement therapy are unlikely to provide an optimal efficacy on both nitric oxide concentration and vasomotion[33,34].

ARTERY INTIMA-MEDIA THICKNESS

Carotid artery intima-media thickness changes can be measured by high-resolution ultrasound and are correlated with carotid and coronary atherosclerosis progression. In women of less than 60 years, estrogen substitution does not seem to have a significant influence on this measurement, but in women over 65 years, the intima-media thickness may become a good marker of the influence of HRT on atherosclerosis[35,36]. However, no study has yet validated this attractive hypothesis.

HEMOSTASIS

After menopause, there is a spontaneous increase in some procoagulant factors such as fibrinogen and factor VII and in anti-fibrinolytic factors such as PAI1. This reflects a tendency towards an increase in thrombotic risk, that HRT is expected to prevent or correct. Oral estrogen substitution tends to decrease fibrinogen and PAI1, but, owing to the first-pass effect, to increase factor VII, fibrinopeptides, fragments 1 and 2 of prothrombin and to decrease anticoagulant factors such as antithrombin III and proteins S and C[37–39]. Thus, in users of oral estrogen substitution, the mean tendency is towards an activation of coagulation fully or partly balanced by fibrinolysis activation with potential increased thrombotic risk in some.

The individual evaluation of risk based only on fibrinogen or PAI1 measurements is misleading, and factor VII, fibrinopeptides and fragments 1 and 2 of prothrombin should also be evaluated. Non-oral administration of estradiol induces only favorable changes in coagulation factors, including factor VII, and in fibrinolytic factors[39]. However, these changes are related to serum estradiol levels, and optimal efficacy on hemostatic balance is obtained only when estradiol reaches concentrations similar to that in the mid-follicular phase. The many users of transdermal systems who do not reach these values can be more easily identified through a serum estradiol evaluation than through a complex and expensive investigation of the hemostatic balance[40].

CONCLUSION

Standardized HRT is far from providing optimal vascular protection to every user and HRT must be customized. During HRT, changes in lipoproteins, glucose metabolism, coagulation, fibrinolysis and arterial function are all expected to participate in cardio-vascular protection and no change is supposed to be detrimental. To verify the optimal adequacy of dose, type and route of administration of steroids in each individual with personal risk profiles, all these changes should theoretically be separately measured. During oral estrogen treatment with or without progestins, the results can be extremely difficult to interpret when both apparently favorable and harmful changes are recorded in the same individual. These include a parallel increase in HDL-C and triglycerides; a parallel decrease in LDL-C and LDL particle size; improvement in fibrinolysis and impairment in coagulation; and vasodilatation and increase in angio-tensinogen. A more consistent and simplified message is obtained with non-oral admini-stration of estradiol. In this case, according to experimental and human data, a serum estradiol level of around 100 pg/ml is the best predictor of a full estrogen-dependent vascular protective effect – on LDL metabolism, the atherosclerosis process, smooth muscle proliferation, repair of vascular injury, hemostatic balance or vasomotion. Associating progesterone, instead of synthetic progestins, also limits the incidence of metabolic and vasomotor disturbances and simplifies individual monitoring. In this case, no side-effect is expected and the only problem is to find the dose adapted to the individual metabolic clearance rate. Then, individual monitoring may be based on serum estradiol levels, which should be within the mid-follicular phase range beyond 60 pg/ml.

References

1. Hemminki E, Sihvo S. A review of posmenopausal hormone therapy recommendations: potential for selection bias. *Obstet Gynecol* 1993;82:1021–8
2. Sturgeon SR, Schairer C, Brinton LA, *et al.* Evidence of a healthy estrogen user survivor effect. *Epidemiology* 1995;6:227–31
3. Barrett-Connor E. The menopause, hormone replacement, and cardiovascular disease: the epidemiologic evidence. *Maturitas* 1996;23:227–34
4. Matthews KA, Kuller LH, Wing RR, *et al.* Prior to use of estrogen replacement therapy, are users healthier than nonusers? *Am J Epidemiol* 1996;143:971–8
5. Rossouw JE. Estrogens for prevention of coronary heart disease. *Circulation* 1996;94:2982–5
6. Gallagher EJ, Viscoli CM, Horwitz RI. The relationship of treatment adherence to the risk of death after myocardial infarction in women. *J Am Med Assoc* 1993;270:742–4
7. Schairer C, Adami HO, Hoover R, *et al.* Cause-specific mortality in women receiving hormone replacement therapy. *Epidemiology* 1997;8:59–65
8. Hemminki E, McPherson K. Impact of postmenopausal hormone therapy on cardiovascular events and cancer: pooled data from clinical trials. *Br Med J* 1997;315:149–53
9. Sidney S, Petitti DB, Quesenberry CP. Myocardial infarction and the use of estrogen and estrogen-progestogen in postmenopausal women. *Ann Intern Med* 1997;127:501–8
10. Daly E, Vessey MP, Hawkins MM, *et al.* Risk of venous thromboembolism in users of hormone replacement therapy. *Lancet* 1996;348:977–80
11. Grodstein F, Stampfer MJ, Goldhaber SZ, *et al.* Prospective study of exogenous hormones and risk of pulmonary embolism in women. *Lancet* 1996;348:983–7
12. Grodstein F, Stampfer MJ, Manson JE, *et al.* Postmenopausal estrogen and progestin use and the risk of cardiovascular disease. *N Engl J Med* 1996;335:453–61
13. Pedersen AT, Lidegaard O, Kreiner S, *et al.* Hormone replacement therapy and risk of non-fatal stroke. *Lancet* 1997;350:1277–83
14. Adams MR, Register TC, Golden DL, *et al.* Medroxyprogesterone acetate antagonizes inhibitory effects of conjugated equine estrogens on coronary artery atherosclerosis. *Arterioscler Thromb Vasc Biol* 1997;17:217–21
15. Barrett-Connor E, Bush TL. Estrogen and coronary heart disease in women. *J Am Med Assoc* 1991;265:1861–7
16. Isles CG, Hole DJ, Hawthorne VM, *et al.* Relation between coronary risk and coronary mortality in women of the Renfrew and Paisley Survey: comparison with men. *Lancet* 1992;339:702–6
17. Kannel WB, Hjortland MC, MacNamara PM, *et al.* Menopause and risk of cardiovascular disease. *Ann Intern Med* 1976;85:447–52
18. Van der Schouw YT, Van der Graaf Y, Steyerberg EW, *et al.* Age at menopause as a risk factor for cardiovascular mortality. *Lancet* 1996;347:714–18
19. Gordon T, Castelli WP, Hjortland MC, *et al.* High density lipoprotein as a protective factor against coronary heart disease. *Am J Med* 1977;62:707–14
20. Eckel RH. Lipoprotein lipase: a multifunctional enzyme relevant to common metabolic diseases. *N Engl J Med* 1989;320:1060–8
21. Margolis S. Diagnosis and management of abnormal plasma lipids. *J Clin Endocrinol Metab* 1990;70:821–5
22. Basdevant A, Blache D, De Lignieres B, *et al.* Hepatic lipase activity during oral and parenteral 17β-estradiol replacement therapy: high-density lipoprotein increase may not be antiatherogenic. *Fertil Steril* 1991;55:1112–17
23. Colvin PL, Auerbach BJ, Case LD, *et al.* A dose-response relationship between sex hormone-induced change in hepatic triglyceride lipase and high-density lipoprotein cholesterol in postmenopausal women. *Metabolism* 1991;40:1052–6
24. Writing Group for the PEPI Trial. Effects of estrogen/progestin regimens on heart disease risk factors in postmenopausal women. *J Am Med Assoc* 1995;273:199–208
25. Nikkila M, Pitkajarvi T, Koivula T, *et al.* Women have a larger and less atherogenic low density lipoprotein particle size than men. *Atherosclerosis* 1996;119:181–190
26. Moorjani S, Dupont A, Labrie F, *et al.* Changes in plasma lipoprotein and apolipoprotein composition in relation to oral versus percutaneous administration of estrogen alone or in cyclic association with Utrogestan in menopausal women. *J Clin Endocrinol Metab* 1991;73:373–9
27. Fletcher CD, Farish E, Dagen MM, *et al.* Short-term changes in lipoproteins and apoproteins during cyclical oestrogen–progestogen replacement therapy. *Maturitas* 1991;14:33–42
28. Wagner JD, Saint Clair RW, Schwenke DC, *et al.* Regional differences in arterial low density lipoprotein metabolism in surgically post menopausal cynomolgus monkeys. Effects of estrogen and progesterone replacement therapy. *Arterioscler Thromb* 1992;12:717–26

29. De Lignieres B. The case for a non plasma lipoproteins etiology of reduced vascular risk in estrogen replacement therapy. *Curr Opin Obstet Gynecol* 1993;5:389–95

30. De Lignieres B. Safety of combined oral contraceptive pills. *Lancet* 1996;347:546

31. Pines A, Fisman EZ, Shapira I, *et al.* Exercise echocardiography in postmenopausal hormone users with mild systemic hypertension. *Am J Cardiol* 1996;78:1385–9

32. Hashimoto M, Akishita M, Eto M, *et al.* Modulation of endothelium-dependent flow-mediated dilatation of the brachial artery by sex and menstrual cycle. *Circulation* 1995;92:3431–5

33. Sullivan JM, Shala BA, Miller LA, *et al.* Progestin enhances vasoconstrictor responses in postmenopausal women receiving estrogen replacement therapy. *Menopause J N Am Menopause Soc* 1995;2:193–9

34. Cicinelli E, Matteo G, Ignarro LJ, *et al.* Acute effects of transdermal estradiol administration on plasma levels of nitric oxide in postmenopausal women. *Fertil Steril* 1997;67:63–6

35. Nabulsi AA, Folsom AR, Szklo M, *et al.* No association of menopause and hormone replacement therapy with carotid artery intima-media thickness. *Circulation* 1996;94:1857–63

36. Espeland MA, Applegate W, Furberg CD, *et al.* Estrogen replacement therapy and progression of intimal-medial thickness in the carotid arteries of postmenopausal women. *Am J Epidemiol* 1995;142:1011–19

37. Lobo RA, Pickar JH, Wild RA, *et al.* Metabolic impact of adding medroxyprogesterone acetate to conjugated estrogen therapy in post-menopausal women. *Obstet Gynecol* 1994;84:987–95

38. Meade TW. Randomised comparison of oestrogen versus oestrogen plus progestogen hormone replacement therapy in women with hysteretomy. *Br Med J* 1996;312:473–8

39. Caine YG, Bauer KA, Barzegar S, *et al.* Coagulation activation following estrogen administration to postmenopausal women. *Thromb Haemost* 1992;68:392–5

40. Lindoff C, Peterson F, Lecander I, *et al.* Transdermal estrogen replacement therapy: beneficial effects on hemostatic risk factors for cardiovascular disease. *Maturitas* 1996;24:43–50

Estrogen deficiency and effect of estrogen replacement therapy on the cardiovascular system

19

G.M.C. Rosano, F. Leonardo and S.L. Chierchia

INTRODUCTION

Recent studies on the cardiovascular effect of ovarian hormones have modified general opinion regarding the cardiovascular implications of hormone replacement therapy after the menopause. From the 1950s to the 1970s, reports showing an increased incidence of coronary artery disease in women who had undergone hysterectomy and oophorectomy suggested the use of estrogen replacement therapy to protect women from atherosclerotic disease[1]. Early findings regarding the cholesterol-lowering effects of estrogens helped to reinforce the opinion that estrogens could provide cardioprotection. However, in the late 1970s findings from the Framingham Heart Study suggested that estrogens increased the risk of cardiovascular disease among menopausal women[2]. At the same time, however, other studies showing cardioprotective effects of estrogens began to be reported and within the last 10 years the Framingham Study has come to stand alone against more than 40 studies which show that estrogen administration after menopause significantly reduces cardiovascular and cerebrovascular morbidity and mortality[3,4]. Recent large-scale epidemiological studies of estrogen use in postmenopausal women and a meta-analysis of the more homogeneous studies indicate an approximately 50% reduction in cardiovascular mortality and morbidity in women taking estrogen replacement therapy as compared to untreated women. These findings are supported by lipid studies indicating that estrogen use raises high-density lipoprotein-cholesterol (HDL-C) and lowers low-density lipoprotein-cholesterol (LDL-C)[5]. It has been initially suggested that most of the cardioprotective effect of estrogen replacement therapy was attributable to favorable changes in the lipid profile. However, recent studies indicated that estrogens have vasoactive properties and may directly influence atheroma formation and suggested that the lipid-lowering effect of the ovarian hormones accounts for not more than 10–20% of the overall cardioprotective effect of estrogens[6,7].

ESTROGENS AND DEVELOPMENT OF ATHEROSCLEROTIC DISEASE

Hormone effects on serum lipids

Total serum cholesterol rises at menopause, with the rise almost entirely due to an increase in LDL-C. Estrogens induce a decrease in total serum cholesterol coupled with an increase in HDL-C and a decrease in LDL-C, while progestins appear to oppose these effects[5]. The HDL/LDL effects are evident with all modes of estrogen administration including oral, transdermal, percutaneous and implant preparations of 17β-estradiol as well as conjugated equine estrogens[8]. One mechanism through which estrogens elevate HDL-C is inhibition of hepatic lipase, the enzyme that destroys HDL-C[9].

Hormone actions in arterial walls

17β-Estradiol and progesterone receptors have been identified in arterial endothelium and smooth muscle cells[10,11]. Direct actions of estrogens on the arterial wall are particularly relevant to current understanding of the processes involved in the development of atherosclerosis. Recent animal studies have reported reduced LDL accumulation and arterial cholesterol ester influx and hydrolysis, inhibition of platelet aggregation, reduced lipoprotein-induced arterial smooth muscle cell proliferation, inhibition of myointimal proliferation associated with mechanical injury or induced by stress, decrease in collagen and elastin production, increase in arterial smooth muscle prostacyclin production and inhibition of foam cell formation[6]. It can be seen that most of the steps involved in the development of atherosclerosis may be inhibited by estrogens. Furthermore, Williams and co-workers[7] have reported that estrogens alone or in combination with progestins inhibited the progression of atherosclerosis in the coronary arteries of cynomolgus monkeys.

Angiographic effects of estrogens

Gruchow and colleagues[12] analyzed the coronary angiograms of 933 women, among whom 16% were taking estrogens at the time of the procedure or within the previous 3 months. Estrogen users had significantly less coronary artery disease than the non-users. The occlusion score increased significantly with age in non-users but not in women taking estrogens. Sullivan and colleagues[13] analyzed coronary arteriograms comparing 1444 women with coronary artery disease (≥ 70% stenosis in at least one artery) and 744 women as controls. Postmenopausal estrogen replacement was found to be a significant protective factor for coronary artery disease. An interesting consideration raised by Sullivan and colleagues' report is that the 744 women who served as controls all underwent coronary angiography because of angina-like chest pain and all had normal coronary angiograms. They represented one-third of all the women having angiograms. The possibility is raised that in some of the women the cardiac symptoms were secondary to ovarian hormone deficiency, as they were in the age group most commonly affected by hot flushes, a symptom of vascular disturbance.

FINDINGS RELATED TO VASOMOTION

Animal studies have shown that the administration of 17β-estradiol leads to an increase in cardiac output, an increase in arterial flow velocity, a decrease in vascular resistance and a decrease in systolic and diastolic blood pressure[14]. Numerous studies have shown that 17β-estradiol induces an increase in blood flow in many different arterial systems including the uterine, urethral, femoral and carotid systems. Human studies have reported estrogen-induced increase in blood flow in the vagina, vulva and uterine and carotid vessels[15,16]. Femoral arteries from rabbits treated with 17β-estradiol showed an enhanced endothelium-dependent relaxation response to acetylcholine[17]. As this effect was not prevented by indomethacin it would appear that a mechanism other than prostacyclin release was responsible for the relaxation response. In addition to the development of atheroma and thrombosis, vessel spasm and changes in arterial tone are of importance in the pathogenesis of ischemic heart disease and myocardial infarction. Recently, it was reported that the coronary vascular response to acetylcholine stimulation in ovariectomized monkeys was increased after 17β-estradiol implants[7]. With the use of quantitative coronary angiography, vasomotor responses to infused acetylcholine were measured and compared in treated and untreated animals. Both groups had been ovariectomized and fed atherogenic diets for 30 months prior to the angiography. Intracoronary infusion of acetylcholine caused constriction in the estrogen-deficient monkeys. Constriction was not seen in the monkeys receiving 17β-estradiol. Instead, minimal dilatation of the left circumflex artery was seen. There was, indeed, lessened atheromatous plaque formation in the estrogen-treated monkeys, but the authors reported that effects on vasomotor response were not related to plaque extent. The authors concluded that estrogens modulate vasomotor responses of atherosclerotic arteries by an endothelium-dependent mechanism, and they speculated that a similar effect may be present in postmenopausal women taking estrogen replacement. Indeed, similar effects have been reported in humans[18,19]. Collins and associates[20] also showed that the reversal of acetylcholine-induced vasoconstriction is gender-dependent, since it was evident only in female patients but not in males. Indeed, acute administration of sublingual 17β-estradiol affects the peripheral vasculature in humans. Volterrani and co-workers[16] showed an increase in forearm blood flow and a reduction in forearm vascular resistance compared to placebo, with no difference in mean arterial blood pressure 40 min after the administration of sublingual 17β-estradiol to postmenopausal volunteers. These results suggest a direct effect of estrogens upon the peripheral vascular system which may involve one or a number of mechanisms, possibly including calcium antagonism or endo-thelium-dependent relaxation. The calcium antagonistic properties of estrogen have been demonstrated in uterine arteries, cardiac myocytes and vascular smooth muscle cells. Since it has been proposed that calcium channel blockers such as nifedipine may reduce the progression of atherosclerosis in animals, it has been suggested that estrogens may reduce the progression of coronary artery disease by a similar mechanism in humans[21,22]. Confirmation of a calcium antagonistic property of estrogens was provided by experiments on isolated guinea-pig cardiac myocytes[23]. 17β-Estradiol at pharmacological doses has a negative inotropic effect on single ventricular myocytes by inhibiting inward calcium current and consequently reducing intracellular free calcium. The calcium antagonistic properties of estrogen may explain the vascular effect of the hormones (i.e. reduction in peripheral vascular resistance) seen in acute and chronic therapy. A calcium antagonistic mechanism may also explain the recently reported reduction in methylergometrine-induced coronary artery constriction after intracoronary administration of 17β-estradiol[24]. 17β-Estradiol may induce vasorelaxation by stimulating endothelium-dependent relaxation, possibly by increasing the release of endothelium-derived relaxing factor (EDRF) or inhibiting calcium influx and therefore causing vasorelaxation. While those mechanisms remain feasible, there appear to be a variety of ways in which the hormone influences vasomotor control. For example, estrogens have effects on the release of epinephrine (adrenaline) and norepinephrine (noradrenaline) at presynaptic junctions. In hypoestrogenic states this control mechanism is disrupted, leading to vasomotor instability as evidenced by sudden increases in serum epinephrine and norepinephrine concentrations when women have hot flushes[25]. Estrogen replacement therapy is extremely effective in restoring vasomotor stability and possibly does so by controlling the release of catecholamines. We have recently shown[26], by means of the study of heart rate variability, that estrogen replacement therapy normalizes the altered neural control of the cardiovascular system in menopausal women. Indeed, an increased sympathetic tone may reduce coronary flow reserve and the normalization of the abnormal control of the cardiovascular system may also be of importance in the cardioprotective effect of the hormones. Estrogens have also been shown to have effects on the release of histamine, 5-hydroxytryptamine, dopamine and vasoactive intestinal peptide[6]. Hyperpolarization of vascular smooth muscle in dog coronary arteries after treatment with 17β-estradiol has led to the suggestion that the hormone acts by increasing K conductance[27].

OTHER EFFECTS RELEVANT TO ESTROGEN CARDIOPROTECTION

The effect of estrogens contained in the birth-control pill preparations upon coagulation has led to the general opinion that estrogens may cause a hypercoagulability state. However, recent studies on hormone replacement regimens have shown that estrogens may favorably affect fibrinolysis, as suggested by the fact that menopausal women taking estrogen replacement therapy have higher levels of plasma fibrinogen compared to premenopausal women. Estrogen replacement therapy is also associated with a reduction of plasma fibrinogen to premenopausal levels[28]. Recent studies have shown that treatment with oral estrogens reduces plasma levels of tissue plasminogen-activator antigen and increases plasma fibrinolytic activity in menopausal women[28]. These findings may help further to explain the mechanism of the protective effect on acute cardiovascular and cerebrovascular ischemic events seen in menopausal women on estrogen replacement therapy. Our group has shown that sublingual 17β-estradiol improves exercise and pacing-induced myocardial ischemia in female patients with coronary artery disease[29]. The improvement of stress-induced myocardial ischemia was of an extent similar to that observed with sublingual nitrates. The anti-ischemic effect of the hormone may be related to both a direct effect upon the coronary vasculature and an effect upon the peripheral vascular resistance. Rosano and co-workers[30] have also recently shown that 17β-estradiol reduces the episodes of chest pain in menopausal patients with syndrome X. These two studies suggest that ovarian hormones may be useful not only for the prevention of cardiovascular events, but also as second line treatment for selected patients with cardiac disorders. It seems that several mechanisms contribute to the cardioprotective effects of estrogens. The importance of changes in lipid profiles has been overestimated in the past. It is now clear that estrogens influence carbohydrate metabolism, positively affect coagulation and have vasoactive properties which are dependent upon their direct and indirect effect upon the different vascular layers.

In conclusion, estrogen deficiency is associated with an increased incidence of cardiovascular mortality and morbidity. This may be related, in part, to an increased progression of coronary atherosclerosis. However, an altered vasomotor tone, the loss of natural calcium antagonism and alteration of the lytic state may also contribute to the rapid rise of cardiovascular events after the menopause. Estrogen replacement therapy reduces the occurrence of cardiovascular disease by positively influencing the development of atherosclerosis, vasomotor tone and the coagulative state.

References

1. Wuest JH, Dry TJ, Edwards JE. The degree of coronary atherosclerosis in bilateral oophorectomized women. *Circulation* 1953;7:801–8
2. Gordon T, Kannel WB, Hjortland MC, *et al.* Menopause and coronary heart disease: the Framingham Study. *Ann Intern Med* 1978;89:157–61
3. Bush TL, Barret-Connor E, Cowan LD, *et al.* Cardiovascular mortality and noncontraceptive use of estrogen in women. *Circulation* 1987;75:1102–9
4. Hunt K, Vessey M, McPherson K, *et al.* Long-term surveillance of mortality and cancer incidence in women receiving hormone replacement therapy. *Br J Obstet Gynaecol* 1987;94:620–35
5. Godsland IF, Wynn V, Crook D, *et al.* Sex, plasma lipoproteins and atherosclerosis: Prevailing assumptions and outstanding questions. *Am Heart J* 1987;114:1467–503
6. Sarrel PM. Effects of ovarian steroids on the cardiovascular system, In Ginsburg J, ed. *Circulation in the Female*. Carnforth, UK: Parthenon Publishing, 1988:117–41
7. Williams JK, Adams MR, Klopfenstein HS. Estrogen modulates responses of atherosclerotic coronary arteries. *Circulation* 1990;81:1680–7

8. Samsioe G. Effects of estrogen in various lipid constituents. *Consultant* 1990;30:58–62

9. Tikkanen M, Nikkala EA, Kuusi T, *et al.* High density lipoprotein-2 and hepatic lipase: reciprocal changes produced by estrogen and norgestrel. *J Clin Endocrinol Metabol* 1982;54:1113–17

10. Horowitz KB, Horowitz LD. Canine vascular tissues are targets for androgens, estrogens, progestins and glucocorticoids. *J Clin Invest* 1982;69:750–8

11. Lin AL, McGill HC, Shain SA. Hormone receptors of the baboon cardiovascular system. *Circ Res* 1982;50:610–16

12. Gruchow HW, Anderson AJ, Barboriak JJ, *et al.* Post-menopausal use of estrogen and occlusion of coronary arteries. *Am Heart J* 1988;115:954–63

13. Sullivan JM, Vander Zwaag R, Lemp GF, *et al.* Postmenopausal estrogen use and coronary atherosclerosis. *Ann Intern Med* 1988;108:358–63

14. Magness RR, Rosenfeld CR. Local and systemic estradiol 17β: effects on uterine and systemic vasodilation. *Am J Physiol* 1989;256:E536–42

15. Killam AP, Rosenfeld CR, Battaglia FC, *et al.* Effect of estrogens on the uterine blood flow of oophorectomized ewes. *Am J Obstet Gynecol* 1973;115:1045–52

16. Volterrani M, Rosano GMC, Coats A, *et al.* Estrogen acutely increases peripheral blood flow in post-menopausal women. *Am J Med* 1995;99:119–22

17. Gisclard V, Miller VM, Vanhoutte PM. Effect of 17β estradiol on endothelium-dependent responses in the rabbit. *J Pharmacol Exp Ther* 1988;244:256

18. Reis SE, Gloth ST, Blumenthal RS. Ethinyl estradiol acutely attenuates abnormal coronary vasomotor responses to acetylcholine in post-menopausal women. *Circulation* 1994;89:52–60

19. Gilligan DM, Quyumi AA, Cannon RO III. Effects of physiological levels of estrogen on coronary vasomotor function in postmenopausal women. *Circulation* 1994;89:2545–51

20. Collins P, Rosano GMC, Sarrel PM, *et al.* Oestradiol 17β attenuates acetylcholine induced coronary arterial constriction in women but not in men with coronary artery disease. *Circulation* 1995;92:24–30

21. Henry PD, Bentley KI. Suppression of atherogenesis in cholesterol fed rabbits treated with nifedipine. *J Clin Invest* 1981;68:1366–9

22. Lichtlen PR, Hugenholtz PG, Hecker H, *et al.* Retardation of angiographic progression of coronary artery disease by nifedipine. *Lancet* 1990;335:1109–13

23. Jiang C, Poole-Wilson PA, Sarrel PM, *et al.* Effect of estradiol 17β on contraction, calcium current and intracellular free calcium in guinea-pig isolated cardiac myocites. *Br J Pharmacol* 1992;106:739–45

24. Rosano GMC, Lopez Hidalgo M, Arie S, *et al.* Acute effect of estradiol 17β upon coronary artery reactivity in menopausal women with coronary artery disease. *Eur Heart J* 1996;17 [Abstr]

25. Kronenberg F, Cote LJ, Linkie DM, *et al.* Menopausal hot flashes: thermoregulatory, cardiovascular and circulating catecholamine and LH changes. *Maturitas* 1984;6:31–43

26. Rosano GMC, Leonardo F, Ponikowski P, *et al.* Estrogen replacement therapy normalizes the autonomic control of the cardiovascular system in menopausal women. *J Am Coll Cardiol* 1996;27:(Suppl A):2 [Abstr]

27. Harder DR, Coulson PB. Estrogen receptors and effects of estrogen on membrane electrical properties of coronary smooth muscle. *J Cell Physiol* 1979;100:375–82

28. Gebara OCE, Mittleman MA, Sutherland P. Association between increased estrogen status and increased fibrinolytic potential in the Framingham Offspring Study. *Circulation* 1995;91:1952–8

29. Rosano GMC, Sarrel PM, Poole-Wilson PA, *et al.* Beneficial effect of estrogen on exercise-induced myocardial ischemia in women with coronary artery disease. *Lancet* 1993;342:133–6

30. Rosano GMC, Lefroy DC, Peters NS, *et al.* Symptomatic response to 17β estradiol in women with syndrome X. *J Am Coll Cardiol* 1998:in press

Differences in clinical and metabolic effects of HRT according to the lengths of the estrogen and progestin phases

20

S.O. Skouby

Estrogen is efficient in relieving the clinical problems of the menopausal syndrome and therefore is the mainstay of hormone replacement therapy (HRT). Continuous estrogen therapy appears to have beneficial effects on cardiovascular risk indicators compared to sequential estrogen administration and combined estrogen/progestin therapy. Some addition of a progestin to the estrogen regimen is recommended to lower the incidence of endometrial hyperplasia and cancer, but no combination of estrogen and progestin has been universally accepted and the doses and types of steroids used in HRT are being continually modified.

The progestins in current use vary from older steroids and natural progesterone and its derivatives to the new third generation progestins such as gestodene and desogestrel. Potential clinical problems with progestin administration are mood disturbances, irregular menstrual bleeding and, causing most concern, attenuation of cardiovascular benefits. Thus, while there are data suggesting a negative impact on blood flow, a blunting of the beneficial effect of estrogen on insulin sensitivity and on biophysical and neuro-endocrine responses to stress, changes in plasma lipids remain the major area of research interest in this regard. The question of whether addition of a progestin to estrogen replacement will diminish the cardio-protective effect, however, will remain open until studies with clinical end-points have been finalized, but combined therapies that minimize the potentially detrimental effects on plasma lipoproteins have now been formulated. The goal of reducing the deleterious progestin effect on the cardioprotection afforded by HRT may also be reached by reducing the frequency of progestin intake or by finding alternatives to systemic treatment. Quarterly use of medroxyprogesterone instead of monthly has been shown to be safe with regard to endometrial hyperplasia and to improve compliance, because of the less frequent menses. An option to decrease the systemic progestin effect is local administration in the uterine cavity. Thus, an intrauterine device (IUD) releasing levonorgestrel marketed for contraceptive purposes has been tested and found to be effective in inducing endometrial protection in perimenopausal women with menopausal complaints.

What is next?

M. Neves-e-Castro

21

After the conclusion of this Symposium there appeared in the literature two articles that may have given rise to some concerns.

One about long-term hormone replacement therapy (HRT) (more than 10 years) and the risk of breast cancer[1]. The other, the HERS trial[2], suggested that HRT for the secondary prevention of cardiovascular diseases might be deleterious during the first year of administration; beneficial effects were only seen after the second year of HRT in patients with heart diseases.

In the first study[1] it is important to emphasize that the trend for HRT, of longer than 10 years duration, reflects only the morbidity and not the mortality. Thus, there is a probability of a higher incidence of diagnosis of breast cancer; however, this does not reflect a higher mortality rate. If these women had not been on HRT they would probably have had a higher morbidity and mortality rate due, among others, to cardiovascular diseases. Thus, it is the net result of HRT that must be taken into consideration by users and physicians when a decision has to be made.

The HERS trial[2] should be interpreted with reservations as to its message for the clinicians. First, the study was performed with one particular combination of estrogens with a progestogen. It refers *only* to this product. Progestational steroids are both chemically and biologically different from one another and are not identical to progesterone. Some of them may adversely modulate the beneficial cardiovascular effects of estrogens. In this context the PEPI trial[3] convincingly showed that only natural progesterone was devoid of such effects. Therefore, the conclusions of the HERS trial cannot be applicable to any effects of estrogens alone (in hysterectomized cardiac patients) or in combination with micronized progesterone. Such studies are very much needed.

The HERS trial seems to suggest that the beneficial effects seen after the second year of HRT are due to genomic-mediated effects on lipids. This is particularly difficult to accept; it is in contrast with many observational and experimental studies which suggest that 70% of the beneficial effects of estrogens in the cardiovascular system are nongenomic and thus, of quick onset. Once an atheromatous plaque is formed it will not disappear when the lipid profile is improved. However a favorable lipid profile may delay its occurrence (primary prevention).

The HERS trial does not give information about the clinical history and autopsy reports of the deceased patients who were on HRT and those in the control group. This lack does not help the interpretation of the results. Therefore, the HERS trial data must be read with caution. For the moment, and until the results of other ongoing trials (WELL-HART) are available there seems to be no need for big changes in the policies applicable to HRT.

Another article has appeared[4] that may be of great help for decision-making taking into account a comprehensive benefit/risk analysis (heart, bone, breast). The heart, the brain, the breast and the uterus are all important targets for estrogen action. They should not be considered independently. They are all parts of the same body; as such, a good HRT regimen is the one that is less harmful and more beneficial for all of them.

References

1. Beral V. The Collaborative Group on Hormonal Factors in Breast Cancer. Breast cancer and hormone replacement therapy: collaborative reanalysis of data from 51 epidemiological studies of 52705 women with breast cancer and 108411 women without breast cancer. *Lancet* 1997; 350:1047–59
2. Hulley SB, *et al.* Randomized trial of estrogen in secondary prevention of coronary heart disease in postmenopausal women. *J Am Med Assoc* 1998;280:605–13
3. The PEPI Writing Group. Effects of estrogen or estrogen/progestin regimens on heart disease risk factors in postmenopausal women. The Postmenopausal Estrogen/Progestin Interventions (PEPI) Trial. *J Am Med Assoc* 1995;273: 199–208
4. Col NF, Eckman MH, Karas RH, *et al.* Patient-specific decisions about hormone replacement therapy in postmeno-pausal women. *J Am Med Assoc* 1997;277:1140–7

Index